HEALTH EDUCATION AND NUTRITION

HEALTH EDUCATION AND NUTRITION

Editor

Amit Sen

ISHA

ISHA BOOKS

Delhi-110033

Health Education and Nutrition

ISBN : 81-8205-238-6

Published in 2005 in India by
Isha Books
D-43, Prithviraj Road,
Adarsh Nagar, Delhi - 110033
e-mail : ishabooks@hotmail.com

Laser Typesetting at : Global Printers, New Delhi
Printed at : Chawla Offset Press, Delhi

Preface

Health, in a living organism, can be understood as homeostasis — the state in which the organism is in balance, with inputs of energy and mass and outputs of energy and mass in approximate equilibrium and the prospects for continued survival of the organism are positive. In humans, with the capacity to analyze and anticipate, health can be understood not only as immediate homeostasis — that is, everything being all right at the moment — but also subjectively as the understanding of the potential of the "healthful" balance being able to continue.

Being healthy is more than not being sick. Nutrition plays an important role in maintaining good health. Nutrition is defined as the science or study of the appropriate diet to promote health. It also refers to the intake of food and other essentials for promoting growth and replacing or repairing worn or damaged tissue. Nutrients support metabolism of all cells thereby sustaining life as we know it. Proper cellular functioning depends on at least 50 essential nutritional compounds and elements. Disease and death may occur if only one of these essential nutrients is deficient or excessive.

Comprehensive health education teaches students fundamental health concepts and skills that foster healthy habits and behaviors for the individual and others through sequential and coordinated teaching of health education, physical education, and family and consumer sciences education at each grade level, kindergarten through grade.

The science and art of health education is eclectic, rapidly evolving, and reflective of an amalgamation of approaches, methods, and strategies from social and health sciences. The range of health education change strategies today is nearly limitless. Health professionals and health education specialists may counsel people at risk for AIDS about safe sex; help children avoid tobacco, alcohol, and drugs; help adults to stop smoking; help patients to manage and cope with their illnesses; and organize communities or advocate policy changes aimed at fostering health improvement.

Health education professionals work all over the world in a variety of settings including schools, worksites, voluntary health organizations, medical settings, and communities. They are challenged to disseminate the best of what is known in new situations. They may also forge and test fundamental theories that drive research and practice in public health, health education, and health care.

The nature, scope and importance of health education are elaborately discussed in the present volume. The basic nutrition concepts and their relationships to health status and disease causation are elaborately narrated.The important nutritional problems and appropriate programmes and policies to address them are also covered. It is hoped the book will prove to be of much use to researchers, planners, governmental and non-governmental agencies, students, teachers, teacher in training and teacher trainers.

Editor

Contents

1

Meaning and Definition of Health

Being healthy is more than not being sick. Nutrition plays an important role in maintaining good health. Identify ways a person can make his/her lifestyle more healthy. Some ideas are listed below:

— Eat a balanced diet.

— Exercise regularly. Aerobic exercise makes our bodies stronger and improves the condition of our hearts.

— Maintain healthy body weight by making correct food choices and exercising regularly.

— Get adequate rest each night.

— Teach other members of your family good nutrition principles.

— Limit foods like candy, soda pop and other nutrient poor foods.

— Make good food choices when eating away from home.

The range of health education and health behavior change strategies today is nearly limitless. Health professionals and health education specialists may counsel people at risk for AIDS about safe sex; help children avoid tobacco, alcohol, and drugs; help adults to stop smoking; help patients to manage and cope with their illnesses; and organize communities or advocate policy changes aimed at fostering health improvement.

Health education professionals work all over the world in a variety of settings including schools, worksites, voluntary health organizations, medical settings, and communities. They are challenged to disseminate the best of what is known in new situations. They may also forge and test fundamental theories that drive research and practice in public health, health education, and health care. A premise of Health Behavior and Health Education is that a dynamic exchange between theory, research, and practice is most likely to produce effective health education.

Perhaps never before have those concerned with health behavior and health education been faced with more challenges and opportunities than they are today. Kanfer and Schefft observed that "as science and technology advance, the greatest mystery of the universe and the least conquered force of nature remains the human being and his actions and human experiences." The body of research in health behavior and health education has grown rapidly over the past two decades, and health education is recognized increasingly as a way to meet public health objectives and improve the success of public health and medical interventions. Although this increasing literature improves the science base of health behavior and health education, it also challenges those in the field to master and be facile with an almost overwhelming body of knowledge.

The science and art of health behavior and health education are eclectic, rapidly evolving, and reflective of an amalgamation of approaches, methods, and strategies from social and health sciences. They draw on the theoretical perspectives, research, and practice tools of such diverse disciplines as psychology, sociology, anthropology, communications, nursing, and marketing.

Health education is also dependent on epidemiology, statistics, and medicine. There is increasing emphasis on identifying evidence-based interventions and disseminating them widely. This often requires individual health education and health behavior professionals to synthesize large and diverse literatures.

Many types of professionals contribute to and conduct health education and health behavior (HEHB) programs and research. Health education practice is strengthened by the close collaboration among professionals of different disciplines, each concerned with the behavioral and social intervention process, and each contributing a unique perspective. Psychology brings to health education a rich legacy of over a hundred years of research and practice on individual differences, motivation, learning, persuasion, and attitude and behavior change.

Physicians are important collaborators and are in key positions to effect change in health behavior. Likewise, nurses and social workers bring to health education their particular expertise in working with individual patients and patients' families to facilitate learning, adjustment, and behavior change, and to improve quality of life. Other health, education, and human service professionals contribute their special expertise as well. Increasingly, there will be partnerships with genetic counselors and other specialists in this rapidly developing field.

Health, Disease, and Health Behavior: The Changing Context

The major causes of death in the United States and other developed countries are now chronic diseases, such as heart disease, cancer, and stroke. Behavioral factors, particularly tobacco use, diet and activity patterns, alcohol consumption, sexual behavior, and avoidable injuries are among the most prominent contributors to mortality. The resurgence of infectious diseases, including foodborne illness and tuberculosis, and the emergence of new infectious diseases such as antibioticresistant infections, HIV/AIDS, Hepatitis C, and human papillomavirus (HPV) are also largely affected by human behaviors.

Substantial suffering, premature mortality, and medical costs can be avoided by positive changes in behavior. Most recently, there has been a renewed focus on public health as a result of anthrax exposure due to terrorism. During the past twenty years, there has been a dramatic increase in public, private, and professional interest in preventing disability and death through changes in lifestyle and participation in screening programs. Much of this interest in disease prevention and early detection has been stimulated by the epidemiologic transition from infectious to chronic diseases as leading causes of death, the aging of the population, rapidly escalating health care costs, and data linking individual behaviors to increased risk of morbidity and mortality.

More recent developments, such as the AIDS epidemic, have also contributed. Even as epidemiologists' efforts to better specify the links between diet, lifestyle, genetic predisposition, and environmental factors and disease approach the limits of science, they continue to generate headlines and influence public policy. Landmark reports in Canada and the United States during the 1970s and 1980s heralded the commitment of governments to health education and promotion. In the United States, federal initiatives for public health education and monitoring populationwide behavior patterns were spurred by the development of the health objectives published in Promoting Health and Preventing Disease: Health Objectives for the Nation and their successors, outlined in Healthy People 2000: National Health Promotion and Disease Prevention Objectives and Healthy People 2010.

Increased interest in behavioral and social determinants of health behavior change spawned numerous training programs and public and commercial service programs. Data systems now make it possible to track trends in risk factors, health behaviors, and healthy environments and policies in the United States and, in some cases, to tie these changes to disease incidence and mortality. Indeed, there have been positive changes in several areas. A major accomplishment has been surpassing the targets for reducing deaths from coronary heart disease and cancer.

Blood pressure control has improved and mean population blood cholesterol levels have declined. Alcohol-related motor vehicle deaths and deaths due to automobile crashes and drowning have continued to decrease. Fewer adults are using tobacco products, and more are engaging in moderate physical activity. More adults are meeting dietary guidelines for consumption of fruits, vegetables, and grain products and for dietary fat as a percentage of calories.

Rates of HIV/AIDS have leveled off and transfusion-related HIV infections have decreased markedly. The proportion of women age fifty and older who have had breast examinations and mammograms has exceeded the goal of 60 percent in forty-seven states. The United States has made progress toward the goal of reducing health disparities for more than half the objectives identified in Healthy People 2000. Major litigation against the tobacco industry and a multistate settlement have resulted in increased restrictions on tobacco advertising and enforcement of laws against selling tobacco to minors. The collective efforts of those in health education and public health have indeed made a difference. While this progress is encouraging, much work remains to be done in these areas. Not all the news is favorable, though. More adults and children are overweight.

Diabetes is increasing in near-epidemic proportions. More adolescents are sexually active. After major increases in seatbelt use in the early 1990s, rates have declined slightly and remain at 67 percent, well below the target rate of 85 percent. One-fifth of children under three years old have not received a basic series of vaccinations for polio, measles, diphtheria, and other diseases. Sixteen percent of adults under sixty-five years of age have no health insurance coverage.

More than 70 percent of adults over age fifty have not been screened for colorectal cancer. Ethnic minorities and those in poverty still experience a disproportionate burden of preventable disease and disability, and for many conditions the gap between disadvantaged and affluent groups is widening.

Changes in the health care system provide new supports and opportunities for health education. Respect for patients' rights is now recognized as fundamental to the practice of medicine. Moreover, there is increased attention to issues of shared decision making. At the same time, patients' access to information about their health care institutions and providers remains limited. Insurance carriers and managed care systems can impose barriers that impede patients' exercise of their rights to make treatment decisions.

The advent of managed health care and health care financing reform pose new challenges as the drive for cost containment affects the entire health care system. While increased accountability often results in cost savings and fewer unnecessary services, little is known about its effects on the health of patients and the overall quality of care. Clinical prevention and behavioral interventions may grow in importance under managed care when their cost-effectiveness is demonstrated and recognized, but the climate of fiscal constraint will probably slow adoption of efficacious behavioral strategies in the short run.

The rapid emergence of new communication technologies and new uses of older technologies, such as the telephone, also provide new opportunities and dilemmas. A new chapter has been added to Health Behavior and Health Education to reflect the importance of new communication technologies. A variety of electronic media for interactive health communication can serve as sources of both general and individualized health information, reminders, and social support for health behavior change. E-health strategies are becoming an important part of the armamentarium of strategies for those in health education and health behavior.

The use of the new technologies be based and evaluated on theories of health behavior. Otherwise, we risk being technology driven instead of outcomes driven. New technologies have the potential to cause harm through misleading or deceptive information, promotion of inappropriate self-care, and interference in the patient-provider relationship. Interactive health communications provide new options for behavioral medicine and preventive medicine and are altering the context of health behavior and health education as they unfold and as their effects are studied.

The Scope and Evolution of Health Education

In the fields of health education and health behavior, the emphasis during the 1970s and 1980s on individuals' behaviors as determinants of health status eclipsed attention to the broader social determinants of health. Advocates of system-level changes to improve health called for renewal of a broad vision of health education and promotion. These calls for moving health education toward social action heralded a renewed enthusiasm for holistic approaches rather than an entirely new worldview. They are well within the tradition of health education and are consistent with its long-standing concern with the impact of social, economic, and political forces on health.

Over the past fifty years, outstanding leaders in health education repeatedly stressed the importance of political, economic, and social factors as determinants of health. The view of health education as an instrument of social change has been renewed and invigorated during the past decade. Policy, advocacy, and organizational change have been adopted as central activities of public health and health education. Most recently, experts have explicitly recommended that interventions on social and behavioral factors related to health should link multiple levels of in-fluence, including the individual, interpersonal, institutional, community, and policy levels.

According to Griffiths, "health education attempts to close the gap between what is known about optimum health practice and that which is actually practiced." Simonds defined health education as aimed at "bringing about behavioral changes in individuals, groups, and larger populations from behaviors that are presumed to be detrimental to health, to behaviors that are conducive to present and future health."

Subsequent definitions of health education emphasized voluntary, informed behavior changes. In 1980, Green defined health education as "any combination of learning experiences designed to facilitate voluntary adaptations of behavior conducive to health. The Role Delineation Project defined health education as "the process of assisting individuals, acting separately or collectively, to make informed decisions about matters affecting their personal health and that of others".

Health education evolved from three settings: communities, schools, and patient care sites. Kurt Lewin's pioneering work in group process and his developmental field theory during the 1930s and 1940s form the intellectual roots of much of today's health education practice.

One of the earliest models developed to explain health behavior, the Health Belief Model, was developed during the 1950s to explain behavior related to tuberculosis screening. Health education includes not only instructional activities and other strategies to change individual health behavior but also organizational efforts, policy directives, economic supports, environmental activities, mass media, and community-level programs.

Two key ideas from an ecologic perspective help direct the identification of personal and environmental leverage points for health promotion and education interventions. First, behavior is viewed as being affected by, and affecting, multiple levels of influence. Five levels of influence for health-related behaviors and conditions have been identified. They are (1) intrapersonal, or individual factors; (2) interpersonal factors; (3) institutional, or organizational factors; (4) community factors; and (5) public policy factors. The second key idea relates to the possibility of reciprocal causation between individuals and their environments; that is, behavior both influences and is influenced by the social environment.

Health education covers the continuum from disease prevention and promotion of optimal health to the detection of illness to treatment, rehabilitation, and long-term care. Health education is delivered in almost every conceivable setting-universities, schools, hospitals, pharmacies, grocery stores and shopping centers, recreation settings, community organizations, voluntary health agencies, worksites, churches, prisons, health maintenance organizations, migrant labor camps, advertising agencies, the Internet, people's homes, and health departments at all levels of government. Health promotion is a term of more recent origin than health education. As defined by Green, it is "any combination of health education and related organizational, economic, and environmental supports for behavior of individuals, groups, or communities conducive to health".

Clearly, health educators have long used more than "educational" strategies. In fact, the terms health promotion and health education are often used interchangeably in the United States. In some countries, such as Australia, health education is considered a much narrower endeavor than health promotion. Nevertheless, although the term health promotion emphasizes efforts to influence the broader social context of health behavior, the two terms remain closely linked and overlapping, share a common historical and philosophical foundation, and are often used in combination.

Health Behavior: A Central Concern of Health Education

The central concern of health education is health behavior. It is included or suggested in every definition of health education and is the crucial dependent variable in most research on the impact of health education intervention strategies. Positive informed changes in health behavior are typically the ultimate aims of health education programs; if behaviors change but health is not subsequently improved, the result is a paradox that must be resolved by examining other issues, such as the link between behavior and health status or the ways in which behavior and health are measured. Informed decision making is a desirable endpoint for problems involving medical uncertainty, and studies suggest that shared decision making may lead to improved patient satisfaction and health outcomes.

Likewise, environmental or structural interventions to change presumed social environmental determinants of health behavior are intended to improve health by changing behavior. Thus, efforts to improve environments, policies, and so on should ultimately be evaluated for their effects on health behavior; if policy changes but it does not lead to measurable changes in behavior, it may be either too weak, too short-lived, or only a limited determinant of behavior. In the broadest sense, health behavior refers to the actions of individuals, groups, and organizations as well as their determinants, correlates, and consequences, including social change, policy development and implementation, improved coping skills, and enhanced quality of life.

This is similar to the working definition of health behavior that Gochman proposed (though his definition emphasized individuals): it includes not only observable, overt actions but also the mental events and feeling states that can be reported and measured. He defined health behavior as: "those personal attributes such as beliefs, expectations, motives, values, perceptions, and other cognitive elements; personality characteristics, including affective and emotional states and traits; and overt behavior patterns, actions, and habits that relate to health maintenance, to health restoration, and to health improvement". There are three categories of health behavior as follows:

— *Preventive health behavior:* Any activity undertaken by an individual who believes himself to be healthy, for the purpose of preventing or detecting illness in an asymptomatic state.

— *Illness behavior:* Any activity undertaken by an individual who perceives himself to be ill, to define the state of health, and to discover a suitable remedy.

— *Sick-role behavior:* Any activity undertaken by an individual who considers himself to be ill, for the purpose of getting well. It includes receiving treatment from medical providers, generally involves a whole range of dependent behaviors, and leads to some degree of exemption from one's usual responsibilities.

During the past century and more specifically during the past few decades, the scope and methods of health education have broadened and diversified dramatically. Today, health education can be found nearly everywhere. The settings for health education are important because they provide channels for delivering programs, provide access to specific populations and gatekeepers, usually have existing communication systems for diffusion of programs, and facilitate development of policies and organizational change to support positive health practices. Six major settings are particularly relevant to contemporary health education: schools, communities, worksites, health care settings, homes, and the consumer marketplace.

Schools: Health education in the schools includes classroom teaching, teacher training, and changes in the school environment that support healthy behaviors. To support long-term health enhancement initiatives, theories of organizational change are used to encourage adoption of comprehensive smoking control programs in schools. Diffusion Theory and the Theory of Reasoned Action have been used to analyze factors associated with adoption of AIDS prevention curricula in Dutch schools.

Communities: Community-based health education draws on social relationships and organizations to reach large populations with media and interpersonal strategies. Models of community organization enable program planners both to gain support for and to design suitable health messages and delivery mechanisms.

Community interventions in churches, clubs, recreation centers, and neighborhoods have been used to encourage healthful nutrition, reduce risk of cardiovascular disease, and use peer influence to promote breast cancer detection among minority women. Worksites. Since its emergence in the mid-

1970s, worksite health promotion has grown and spawned new tools for health educators. Because people spend so much time at work, the workplace is both a source of stress and a source of social support.

Effective worksite programs can harness social support as a buffer to stress, with the goal of improving worker health and health practices. Today many businesses, particularly large corporations, provide health promotion programs for their employees. Both high-risk and populationwide strategies have been used in programs to reduce the risk of cancer and cardiovascular disease.

Health education for high-risk persons, patients, their families, and the surrounding community and inservice training for health care providers are all part of health care today. The changing nature of health service delivery has stimulated greater emphasis on health education in physicians' of-fices, health maintenance organizations, public health clinics, and hospital. Primary care settings, in particular, provide an opportunity to reach a substantial number of people. Health education in these settings focuses on preventing and detecting disease, helping people make decisions about genetic testing, and managing acute and chronic illnesses.

Homes: Health behavior change interventions are delivered to people in their homes, both through traditional public health means-home visits-and through a variety of communication channels and media such as the Internet, telephone, and mail. The use of strategies such as mailed tailored messages and motivational interviewing by telephone makes it possible to reach larger groups and high-risk groups in a convenient way that reduces barriers to their receiving motivational messages.

The Consumer Marketplace: The advent of home health and self-care products, as well as the use of "health" appeals to sell consumer goods, has created new opportunities both for health education and for misleading consumers about the potential health effects of items they can purchase. Social marketing, with its roots in consumer behavior theory, is used increasingly by health educators to enhance the salience of health messages and to improve their persuasive impact.

Theories of Consumer Information Processing (CIP) provide a framework for understanding why people do or do not pay attention to, understand, and make use of consumer health information such as nutrient labels on packaged food products.

For health education to be effective, it should be designed with an understanding of the recipients, or target audiences, and their health and social characteristics as well as their beliefs, attitudes, values, skills, and past behaviors. These audiences consist of people who may be reached as individuals, in groups, through organizations, as communities or sociopolitical entities, or through some combination of these. They may be health professionals, clients, people at risk for disease, or patients. There are four dimensions in which the potential audiences can be characterized: sociodemographic characteristics, ethnic or racial background, life cycle stage, and disease or at-risk status.

Socioeconomic status has been linked with both health status and health behavior, with less affluent persons consistently experiencing higher morbidity and mortality. The recognition of differences in disease and mortality rates across socioeconomic and ethnic or racial groups has led to increasing efforts to reduce or eliminate such health disparities. For example, it has long been known that African Americans die at earlier ages than do whites. As of 1998, life expectancy for African American males was 67.6 years compared to 74.5 years for white males. The difference is slightly less for African American women, 74.8 versus 80 for white women, but still alarmingly discrepant.

A variety of sociodemographic characteristics such as gender, age, race, marital status, place of residence, and employment characterize health education audiences. These factors, while generally not modifiable within the bounds of health education programs, are useful in guiding the tailoring of strategies and educational material and identifying channels through which to reach consumers. Printed educational materials should be appropriate to, and, ideally, tailored to the educational and reading levels of particular target audiences and be consistent with their ethnic and cultural backgrounds.

Life Cycle Stage: Health education is provided for people at every stage of the life cycle, from childbirth education, the beneficiaries of which are not yet born, to self-care education and rehabilitation for the very old. Developmental perspectives help guide the choice of intervention and research methods. Children may have misperceptions about health and illness, such as that illnesses are a punishment for bad behavior.

Knowledge of children's cognitive development helps provide a framework for understanding these beliefs and ways to respond to them. Adolescents may feel invulnerable to accidents and chronic diseases. The Health Belief Model is a useful framework for understanding the factors that may predispose youth to engage in unsafe sexual practices. Older adults may attribute symptoms of cancer to the inexorable process of aging. Beliefs such as this must be considered in designing, implementing, and evaluating health education programs.

Disease and At-Risk Status: People who are diagnosed with specific diseases often experience not only symptoms but also the distress associated with their prognosis and with having to make decisions about medical care. Thus, while they may benefit from receiving health education, their ability to attend to new information may be compromised at critical points due to their illness. Because of this, the timing, channels, and audiences for patient education need to be carefully considered. Successful patient education depends on a sound understanding of the patient's view of the world.

For individuals at high risk due to family history or identified risk factors, health behavior change interventions may have heightened salience when linked to strategies for reducing individual rise. Even so, strategies used to enable initial changes in behavior, such as quitting smoking, may be insufficient for maintaining behavior change over the long term even in these persons. Models and theories of health behavior can suggest strategies for relapse prevention for high-risk individuals.

Health Promotion and Health Behavior Research

Over the past two decades, research programs have been established to identify and test the most effective methods for achieving health behavior change. More precise quantification of personal health behaviors and improved health outcomes has grown from partnerships between behavioral health scientists and biomedical experts. During this period, findings from some major health behavior intervention studies have become available and have provided important insights for the field.

In the late 1970s and early 1980s, three large community cardiovascular disease intervention studies were begun in California, Minnesota, and Rhode Island. Each study addressed smoking, hypertension, high-fat diets, obesity, and physical inactivity-all widespread risk factors that many practitioners were tackling. The multicomponent risk reduction programs in these trials used mass media, interpersonal education programs for the public, professionals, and those at high risk. Community organization strategies were used to create institutional and environmental support for the programs, and theory-derived program planning strategies emphasized community participation.

The challenge of understanding and improving health behavior is a central challenge for health policy today, and is "one of the most complex tasks yet confronted by science. To competently address that challenge, the . . . research community must simply do more and do it better" in certain key areas of behavioral research. A coordinated and focused effort will be essential to resolving many of the most vexing health issues facing our society. The integration of the best available knowledge from theory, research, and health promotion and education practice can help advance that agenda in the next decade.

2

Meaning, Definition, Objectives and Principles of Health Education

A Cross-Cultural Comparison of Health Promoting Behaviour

It has been a consistent goal of epidemiological research to identify specific behaviors that contribute to a variety of both negative and positive health outcomes, and to describe the underlying determinants of those behaviors. Such knowledge can then be used by health educators to improve health outcomes by implementing programs that attempt to eliminate risky behaviors and promote positive ones. In searching for the determinants of personal health behaviors, much of the focus in the past has been on the individual (or micro) level. Such constructs as locus of control, self-esteem, loneliness, depression, hardiness, resilience, and personality type have been used to explain individual behavior patterns.

At the same time, health behaviors that are prevalent within larger populations may have determinants that go beyond individual variables. As such, there is growing interest in the macro level determinants of health behavior including the role of social norms, culture, mass media, national health policies, advertising practices, physical and social environments, etc. Comprehensive behavior change interventions of the future will likely be most effective if they are able to address both the micro and macro level determinants of behavior.

Findings are based on a convenience sample of 1,233 college students aged 18 years and older who were attending one of two institutions in the western US, or an institution in central Japan. Participants were taken from large sections of general education courses. Almost all students at Brigham Young University, and approximately 50% at Utah State University, are members of the Church of Jesus Christ of Latter-day Saints. As such, the U.S. sample represents a unique population in terms of religious affiliation and spiritual orientation that is not representative of other U.S. college populations with respect to religiosity and spirituality.

In order to quantify the degree to which a variety of health promoting behaviors are practiced among certain groups, a number of health behavior surveys have been developed including the Health-Promoting Lifestyle Profile (HPLP). The HPLP was designed to assess the relationship between several different lifestyle behaviors and health status. The questionnaire has a 4-point response format with 70 items that are divided into six subscales: health responsibility, spiritual growth, physical activity, nutrition, interpersonal support, and stress management.

A total HPLP score provides a comprehensive measure of health promoting lifestyles. Previous evaluation of the HPLP indicates that the scale is both valid and reliable with an initial Cronbach's alpha rating of .92 indicating high internal consistency, and test-retest reliability above .85 indicating acceptable levels of stability. Content and face validity were initially established using expert reviews and extensive pilot tests. In 2000, the HPLP was translated into Japanese and evaluated for validity and reliability. After pilot testing, the HPLP was given to 337 participants in northern Japan. Cronbach's alphas of .94 and .91 were obtained respectively at initial testing and at retesting two weeks later.

Researchers concluded that the instrument was valid, reliable, culturally relevant, and capable of describing the health-promoting components of lifestyle among Japanese respondents. Approval from institutional review boards at participating institutions was obtained. After receiving appropriate instructions, course instructors administered the survey to students. Voluntary participation based on informed consent yielded student response rates of approximately 80-90 percent in each of the surveyed courses. English and Japanese versions of the HPLP were used to collect the data in the US and Japan respectively. Data was hand entered into an excel file by research assistants and then each entry was rechecked to ensure accuracy.

Differences between US and Japanese responses to categorical questions (weight loss, eating disorders, and exercise) were assessed using the chi-square test. Differences in the mean level of agreement to HPLP subscale statements (involving interpersonal relations, nutrition, health responsibility, exercise, stress management, and spiritual growth), and a summary HPLP score, were compared between the US and Japan using the t-test.

The normality assumption was reasonably satisfied for the HPLP and for each subscale according to the Kolmogorov-Smirnov test. Equality of variances were assessed using an F statistic. Pooled variances or the Satterthwaite variance was used in computing the t statistic, depending on whether the assumption of equal variances was satisfied. All analyses were stratified by gender. The linear association between HPLP and variables related to weight loss, eating disorders, exercise, and select demographics (age, education, and gender) was assessed using multiple regression analysis.

Analysis was based on 594 respondents residing in the US (249 men, 343 women, and 2 undeclared), and 629 respondents residing in Japan (62 men, 564 women, and 3 undeclared). The average age was 21.0 in the US (22.0 for men and 20.2 for women), and 21.5 in Japan (22.2 for men and 21.4 for women). Although all respondents in the sample had at least a high-school degree, men and women in Japan were significantly more likely to have a two- or four-year college degree.

Men in the US compared with Japan were significantly less likely to diet to lose weight but more likely to exercise on almost a daily basis. Japanese men were more likely to indicate they are unsure whether they currently or previously had an eating disorder. Because of the high level of this response among men, we were not able to evaluate whether a history of eating disorders differed between men in the US and Japan. Women in the US were significantly more likely than women in Japan to be currently trying to lose weight and to exercise on almost a daily basis. They were also more likely to have had an eating disorder. Yet the stated importance of losing weight and the frequency of dieting to lose weight was higher among Japanese women.

A comparison between men and women shows that issues related to weight are of greater importance for women than men in both countries. Respondents were asked to indicate the frequency with which they engaged in each behavior, with higher scores representing a greater level of participation. Mean responses to nutrition and health responsibility were higher for both women and men in Japan, and mean exercise and spiritual growth were higher for both women and men in the US. Total HPLP scores were higher for both men and women in the US versus men and women in Japan, although statistical significance was achieved only for differences between women.

For US respondents, HPLP scores were significantly lower for men, and lower for those who thought it was important to lose weight and who currently had an eating disorder. On the other hand, HPLP scores were significantly higher for those who exercised at least 4-5 times per week. For Japanese respondents, HPLP scores were also significantly lower for men. HPLP scores were significantly higher, however, for those who felt that weight loss was somewhat important or always on their mind, those who exercised, and those who were older.

Health Responsibility

The health responsibility subscale measures the degree to which respondents actively seek reliable health care information from health providers, and the degree to which they engage in positive self-care practices such as self-examinations. Low nutrition scores for the US participants is not surprising given that skipping meals, frequent snacking, and indulgence in fast foods seem to be common practices in the US. Such dietary practices are generally thought to be a primary cause of rising rates of obesity. At present, Asian cultures may be somewhat health protective in terms of honoring traditional diets that are high in grains and vegetables while maintaining nutritional norms that somewhat limit snacking, skipping meals, and other poor nutritional practices.

Asian students who migrate to the US for higher education tend to have diets that are superior to their American classmates in terms of diet composition and eating habits. Yet the longer that these students resided in the US the more likely they were to skip meals, indulge in high fat/sugar snacks, and select fast foods when they ate out. Likewise, changes in the social environment in Japan may be leading to diets that include more snacking, fast foods, and high fat/high sugar diets.

US participants were more likely to outperform the Japanese in terms of active lifestyles. A higher HPLP subscale score in this area was confirmed by actual reports of activity levels among students. Almost half of American women (48%) reported exercising at least four times per week, but only 17% of Japanese women indicated similar levels of activity. In spite of lower exercise scores, it may be possible that in Japan the levels of activity involved in commuting (including walking and bicycling) may somewhat counterbalance the low levels of reported exercise. It is possible that for many US men and women the goal of exercise is to enhance appearance and social acceptance, rather than improve physical health.

Given their higher scores on the health responsibility subscale, it is possible that exercise for Japanese students is pursued more for health enhancement than for concerns over appearance. If so, appearance and social acceptance may be stronger motivations for exercise than simply improved health status (as in Japan). However, indicate that higher levels of activity correlate significantly with higher total HPLP scores for both US and Japanese students, regardless of underlying motivation. Similarly, research in Japan has reported that high levels of leisure-time physical activity tend to accompany other healthy behaviors.

Weight Management

Not surprisingly, it was found that concerns over weight management were greater for women than for men in both cultures. Paradoxically, college women in Japan were more likely to rate weight loss as "very important" or "always on my mind" as compared with their US counterparts (47% vs. 36%). Yet more American women were actively trying to lose weight at the time of the survey (57% vs. 41%) and had experienced eating disorders in the past (19% vs. 12%). Even though the majority of US women were trying to lose weight, it is possible that positive statements about weight loss importance may be considered undesirable by members of this group, and may even indicate an unhealthy preoccupation. This theory is supported by the finding that statements indicating that weight loss is important were negatively correlated with overall HPLP scores for US Students. Yet the reverse was true for Japanese participants. Given the somewhat higher health responsibility scores for the Japanese, and their already very low levels of overweight, it is possible that Japanese students rated weight loss as being important because of positive health considerations related to healthy weight management. In support of this possibility, the multivariate regression analysis found that for Japanese students, statements that weight loss was "somewhat important" or "always on my mind" were positively correlated with overall HPLP scores.

Alternatively, it is also possible that the Western preoccupation with thinness as the only acceptable body type may be creeping into Japanese culture and contributing to unnecessary concerns about weight loss and dieting. Half of American women reported dieting at least once a year, whereas over 80% of Japanese women stated that they diet at that level. While past research suggests lower rates of eating disorders among Japanese women, the relatively high rates of dieting and the high importance of weight loss found among the Japanese women may indicate a negative move toward unhealthy dieting practices that are motivated by social pressure rather than health.

While the motivation for exercise among US women is still uncertain (appearance vs. health), the From a cultural standpoint, Japanese college students may be more receptive to positive nutrition and fitness messages that focus on health responsibility and self-care independence than their US counterparts. At the same time, this population seems to be at risk for succumbing to Western ideals that support unrealistic body images and that promote restrictive dieting practices as normative behaviors for managing weight and enhancing appearance.

Likewise, Japanese nutritional practices are at risk of being negatively impacted by a growing fast food culture that is fueled by Western media. Before eating disorders, poor nutritional habits, and unhealthy dieting practices reach levels similar to the US, there seems to be a window of opportunity for comprehensive health education interventions that can protect positive practices while curtailing the spread of negative influences.

South Korea has been successful at the national level in supporting messages and policies that favor traditional, and more nutritious, diets-thereby using macro level interventions to support those elements of the culture that are already health protective. The result has been lower levels of fat intake and less obesity in South Korea as compared with other Asian countries. Similarly, Japan may be in a position to bolster positive nutrition practices through national policies and education programs that counter the growing efforts of the fast food industry to make burgers and fries the foundation of a new national diet.

One of the greatest disparities found in in the area of exercise, with Japanese students engaging in relatively low levels of purposeful physical activity. While activity associated with commuting (e.g. walking, bicycling) may diminish this difference, there is an opportunity to evaluate exercise opportunities for activity available to college students, and to create social environments and physical facilities that support exercise.

Using multivariate regression analysis, found a significant correlation between overall HPLP scores and increased levels of exercise among Japanese students. This relationship between exercise and overall healthy lifestyles might be exploited more effectively through increased levels of national fitness promotion. Beyond health enhancement, there is also an opportunity to promote exercise as a sustainable method for weight management that is preferable to restrictive dieting. If not redirected, the high levels of restrictive dieting reported by Japanese students in may soon lead to levels of eating disorders similar to those reported in the US.

In relation to weight management, proper nutrition, and fitness, one of the primary challenges facing health education is the confusion created by having two sets of potentially conflicting goals. For the health educator, the goal is the promotion of holistic health. For those individuals who are targeted by health education programs, on the other hand, the goal is often the pursuit of a more attractive body-even if health is compromised in the process.

At present, Japan seems to have an edge in relation to higher levels of health responsibility and nutrition. Even so, the excessive concern over weight loss and the high prevalence of restrictive dieting found and it may indicate that the Japanese are adopting Western standards of beauty, and are pursuing potentially unhealthy methods of weight management. While the US participants scored higher on exercise and spirituality subscales, they still seem to be preoccupied with the pursuit of unrealistic body ideals.

The majority of women were trying to lose weight, and one out of five indicated experience with an eating disorder. Health responsibility and nutrition scores reflected room for improvement, a finding that is supported elsewhere in the literature. On a positive note, the weight management efforts are shifting from a reliance on restrictive dieting, to a more balanced approach that includes higher levels of exercise. This trend should be supported and at the same time enhanced by health education messages that encourage a more balanced, holistic perspective in relation to the positive role of exercise.

Given conflicting goals (appearance vs. health), there is a need for leadership from the health education profession in developing and promoting common goals in a variety of diverse cultural settings. For example, health education is in a position to help fight against the notion that only very thin bodies are socially acceptable. There is growing evidence that high levels of health and happiness can be achieved at many different body sizes. In promoting positive nutrition practices, health educators can develop coalitions, lobby politicians, propose national policies, and develop mass media messages that counter fast food and junk food advertising, and that support the availability, accessibility, affordability, and desirability of healthy food choices. The US sample may have been even less representative of American university students due to the unique religious affiliation of most participants. As such, the generalizability of results is weakened. Future research should include a wider diversity of participants.

In order to be effective behavior change agents, health educators need to develop comprehensive interventions that address both the micro and macro level determinants of health behaviors. The differences in health promoting lifestyle behaviors between two diverse populations from the larger perspective of culture and social environment. While the analysis does not allow for cause and effect determinations, it does offer potential insights that might be useful in guiding the development of comprehensive interventions. It seems probable that population based interventions that recognize and support cultural strengths, while resisting weaknesses, will be more successful than those that fail to take such a broad perspective.

Food Safety: An International Public Health Issue

Foodborne disease caused by microbial pathogens remains a significant international public health problem in the 21st century, so much so that governments spanning the globe are intensifying their efforts to improve food safety. In the U.S., one of the priorities in the Healthy People 2010 initiative focuses on food safety. In addition, a new guideline, 'keeping food safe to eat', was added to the 2000 edition of the Dietary Guidelines for Americans. The WHO recently announced a plan to expand its food safety program globally, regionally, and nationally. Headline news stories focusing on widespread outbreaks of foodborne illness on virtually every continent are vivid reminders that the food that nourishes and sustains us also can be debilitating, and in some cases, deadly.

In fact, "food is the major source of exposure to pathogenic agents...from which no one in either developing or developed countries is spared". Although the incidence of foodborne illness is difficult to determine, the WHO estimates that worldwide there are thousands of millions cases of foodborne illnesses annually and over two million children die from these diseases each year. In developed nations, the WHO estimates that a third of the population has a foodborne illness event yearly accounting for about 20 million deaths. Recently, the Centers for Disease Control and Prevention estimated that 5,000 deaths and 325,000 hospitalizations each year in the United States are food-related. In the U.S., hospital costs for treating victims of foodborne illnesses likely top $3 billion and lost productivity costs amount to as much as $9 billion. In

England and Wales, the estimated medical costs and value of lives lost from just 5 foodborne illnesses are £300 to 700 million annually. None of the cost estimates include the total societal burden of chronic, long-term consequences of some foodborne illnesses.

These estimates also do not account for the vast majority of foodborne disease cases caused by mishandling of food at home that go unreported because consumers believe they have the 'flu'. In addition, the costs do not reflect the devastating impact foodborne illness can have on a country's economy. For instance, the 1991 cholera epidemic in Peru resulted in the loss of $700 million in fish exports. FoodNet, a new active surveillance program, is helping to more accurately gather information about foodborne illness incidence and the actual burden of foodborne pathogens.

The importance of foodborne illness as a current public health concern is underscored by the increasing numbers of 'at risk' or highly susceptible populations. The number of people in the U.S. considered at increased risk for foodborne illness is now estimated to equal one-fourth of the population. In developing countries, the percent of the population at increased risk for foodborne illness may be even higher due to effects of malnutrition such as reduced immune system function. Those considered 'at risk' include persons with weakened immune systems due to disease (e.g., HIV/AIDS) or pharmaceutical or radiological treatments; pregnant women and their fetuses; lactating mothers; infants and young children; preschool children in day care; and elderly persons.

Others who may be at a disproportionately greater risk include those living in institutional settings and financially disadvantaged individuals such as those who are homeless, migrants, displaced, or refugees. Many consumers are unaware that some people are at higher risk of foodborne disease than others are—and if they are aware of risk groups, they often fail to recognize when they belong to a risk group. The discovery of pathogenic microbes not previously known to cause foodborne illness along with the emergence of antibiotic resistant strains of foodborne pathogens further highlights the importance of this public health concern.

Today, we are aware of over 5 times more foodborne pathogens than we were just 50 years ago. These pathogenic microbes have made cooking and eating practices that were once consider safe, like eating rare ground beef or raw eggs, particularly dangerous because it's difficult to convince consumers that it's no longer safe to continue a behavior when they feel they have 'always done it and never gotten sick'. Medically treated cases of foodborne illnesses caused by new pathogens are frequently underreported and nearly half of all recorded foodborne illnesses are of unknown cause. Technological and societal changes over the last quarter century also have contributed to the opportunities for foodborne disease caused by mishandling of food and cross-contamination.

Food today is more extensively processed, is handled at more steps between farm and table, and is stored and transported for longer periods than in the past, and these extra steps create opportunities for microbial contamination. In industrialized countries eating occasions have proliferated. Considering that each person in the U.S. eats, on average, at least four times daily, there could be a billion opportunities each day for someone to transmit and/or contract a foodborne disease.

The foods we eat and where we eat them have changed, too. Expanding urban migration and increased dependence on stored foods coupled with insufficient access to safe water and sanitary food preparation facilities present important food safety obstacles in many developing nations. The convenience-driven lives of many Westernized countries, which compels many to stash food unrefrigerated in the car, sports-bag, or desk drawer to be eaten on the run later presents other food safety hazards.

Both the U.S. and U.K. educational systems once taught food safety in family and consumer sciences (home economics) classes in virtually every secondary school. Changes over the past decade have resulted in a reduction or even elimination of such courses. Increasing numbers of working mothers and growing reliance on frozen meals, restaurant dining, and take-out foods have decreased opportunities for many children to learn safe food handling via observation. As a result, a large proportion of individuals have limited food preparation experience, have never learned basic principles of food safety, and, thus, lack the critical knowledge needed to help them proactively protect themselves and their families.

Indeed, the National Academy of Sciences' report Ensuring Safe Food: From Production to Consumption identified major areas where the current U.S. food safety system falls short—one of these areas is limited consumer knowledge. Additionally, one of the seven food safety goals of the Healthy People 2010 is to increase the proportion of consumers who follow key food safety practices. The WHO also has cited food safety education as a key health improving strategy for the entire world. Gro Harlem Brundtland, WHO Director-General stated that "more needs to be done globally to reverse the upward curve which represents escalating sickness and death from consumption of unsafe food". To help curtail the high rate and exorbitant cost of foodborne disease, both WHO and U.S. government agencies (i.e., USDA, FDA) have called for the integration of food safety concepts into health education programs for consumers and school age children. Education is one of the most critical interventions in the prevention of foodborne illness.

Although a natural fit in the health curriculum, traditionally, health education curricula, textbooks, and journals have given scant attention to the prevention of foodborne illness even though they often address prevention of other infectious diseases, such as common infections (e.g., colds and influenza) and sexually transmitted diseases.

Major Foodborne Pathogens

A wide variety of agents are capable of causing infectious

foodborne illness in humans including bacteria, viruses, molds, parasites, and infectious protein-containing particles that may be prions. Noninfectious causes of foodborne illnesses (e.g., heavy metals [e.g., copper, zinc, tin, cadmium, mercury], poison mushrooms [e.g., amatoxins, phallotoxins], chemicals [e.g., histamine, the causative agent in scombroid fish poisoning], and nonbacterial toxins [e.g., toxins produced by dinoflagellates that cause paralytic shellfish poisoning and ciguatera] are relatively rare, accounting for less than two percent of all foodborne illnesses in the U.S. and beyond the scope of this article.

Bacterial Foodborne Illnesses

Bacteria are everywhere in nature. They are found in the food we eat, the water we drink, and air we breathe. They live in our intestines, on our skin, in the refrigerator, and on kitchen countertops. Most are harmless, some have beneficial effects, as in the aging of cheeses, but a few are pathogenic and can cause illness. While bacteria are ubiquitous in the environment, most of the pathogenic bacteria that cause foodborne illness originate in an infected human or animal and reach food by one of three fairly well-defined routes.

Contamination by feces

Many foodborne illness bacteria are excreted abundantly in the feces of infected humans or animals. In countries with inadequate sanitation, the water used for drinking, cooking, washing produce and dishes, and fishing is frequently contaminated with sewage and is a major source of illness. Similarly, farmers in these countries may use untreated sewage or animal feces as fertilizer, thus contaminating crops in the field. In the U.S. and other industrialized countries, fecal contamination usually occurs when food is handled by a person who has come in contact with feces or sewage (as in using the bathroom or changing diapers) and has not thoroughly washed his or her hands. Just one gram of fecal matter from an infected person may contain a trillion bacteria —an infectious dose for Salmonella or Vibrio Cholerae. But, as few as 10 to 100 Shigella bacteria can produce infection. Insects, such as houseflies, also may carry bacteria from sewage to food. Foodborne illnesses that are acquired from fecal matter in one of these ways are sometimes said to be transmitted by the fecal-oral route.

Contamination by an infected individual

Some pathogenic bacteria can be transferred to food directly by an infected individual. For example, a food handler who has an open wound or who coughs or sneezes onto food may contaminate the food. Pets also may be a source of foodborne pathogens that can contaminate food via the unwashed hands of food preparers.

Cross-contamination

Cross-contamination occurs when bacteria present in one food are transferred to another food. This may occur when an uncontaminated food touches a contaminated food or any object, such as a plate, knife, or cutting board, which came in contact with contaminated food. For instance, let's say a person sliced raw chicken contaminated with pathogenic bacteria and then sliced lettuce that was not contaminated. After slicing the chicken, the cutting board, knife, and his or her hands also were contaminated with bacteria that will spread to the lettuce if these items are not thoroughly washed before slicing the lettuce. While the bacteria on the chicken will be killed when it is cooked, the lettuce doesn't get cooked and the bacteria can grow if the lettuce is held at a suitable temperature. All bacteria can be transferred to food via cross-contamination.

How bacteria cause foodborne illness. There are two ways in which pathogenic bacteria can cause disease. Some bacterial cells, such as C. jejuni, Salmonella, Listeria monocytogenes, and E. coli, injure the body directly by causing a foodborne infection. Others damage the body with a toxin that they produce and release. Staphylococcus aureus, Clostridium perfringens, Clostridium botulinum, and other toxin-producing bacteria cause foodborne intoxications. Unlike foodborne infections, live bacteria need not be present in food for a foodborne intoxication to occur. Toxin-producing bacteria need only to have, at some point, infused the food with their toxin.

Campylobacter jejuni: C. jejuni is a problem worldwide. It is recognized as a major public health problem in northern European countries, North America, New Zealand, and Australia. In the U.S. and U.K., it is the most common cause of bacterial diarrhea with millions suffering infections yearly. Raw or undercooked protein rich foods of animal origin, particularly poultry and raw milk, are the main vehicles that carry this pathogen into the human body. Meat becomes infected with C. jejuni mainly when processing procedures or equipment rupture an animal's intestinal tract and cause fecal matter to contaminate the raw flesh. In the U.S., food safety laws require that animal flesh contaminated with fecal matter be trimmed away and discarded and/or cleansed, depending on the type of animal. Raw milk can become contaminated with C. jejuni either from feces that accidentally get into the milk or infected cow udders. C. jejuni also can be spread to other foods by other routes of fecal contamination and cross-contamination. Temperatures below 32°F (0°C) or above 165°F (74°C) destroy C. jejuni. Thus, infection can be prevented by thoroughly cooking or freezing raw protein-rich foods of animal origin, and pasteurizing milk.

Salmonella: Salmonella has been recognized as a pathogen for humans and animals for more than a century. In the last decade, many countries throughout the world experienced an upsurge in the number of Salmonella infections. Although nontyphoidal Salmonella is a major problem in industrialized countries, Salmonella Typhi (the bacterium that causes typhoid fever) is uncommon. Salmonella infection is often traced to raw or undercooked poultry and eggs, raw milk, and produce, particularly melons that came in contact with contaminated soil or water. Salmonella bacteria, like C. jejuni, are commonly found in animal fecal matter and can be spread to animal flesh during processing as well as to raw milk. A strain of

Salmonella appearing in chickens can infect the hen's internal organs and be present in the yolk when the egg is laid. Salmonella can grow rapidly on the surface of produce and when a knife cuts through the skin or rind, it can transfer some of the bacteria from the outside to the part we eat. Salmonella also spreads via other routes of fecal contamination and cross-contamination.

All of the over 2200 types of Salmonella bacteria can be killed by thoroughly cooking animal flesh and eggs and pasteurizing milk. The risk of infection from raw produce can be minimized by sanitary food handling procedures including thoroughly washing produce before preparing or eating it. Once produce is sliced, it should be eaten immediately or refrigerated. In just four hours, bacteria on a sliced melon left at room temperature can multiply to dangerous levels.

Escherichia coli: Although most types of E. coli bacteria are harmless inhabitants of the human intestinal tract, some types are major causes of diarrhea worldwide and at least six types are known to cause serious illness. Fortunately, the rate of serious E. coli infections is relatively low. However, in 1993, one of the dangerous types, E. coli 0157:H7 caused one of the most serious outbreaks of foodborne illness in the U.S. This bacterium infected more than 500 people and killed four children in western states, most of whom had eaten undercooked hamburgers at local fast food restaurants. It was this outbreak that led to the food safety handling instructions labels now required on fresh meats. This bacterium causes illness by attaching itself to the intestinal wall and then producing a toxin. In severe cases, the intestinal wall becomes so damaged that the toxin can leak into the person's bloodstream, spread to vital organs and damage them so severely that death results. Undercooked meat is the most frequent cause of this infection. Raw milk, unwashed produce, and unpasteurized, unpreserved apple cider are other common culprits. E. coli 0157:H7 is found in the intestinal tracts of cattle and is harmless to the animals. Like C. jejuni and Salmonella, it contaminates meat if, during slaughter, fecal matter spills onto the carcass. E. coli 0157:H7 can be transmitted to other foods by other sources of fecal contamination as well as by cross-contamination.

E. coli 0157:H7 can survive freezer temperatures and can multiply slowly at temperatures as low as 44°F (7°C). Thoroughly cooking meat to 160°F (70°C) and pasteurization are the best safeguards against infection. Illness can be minimized by thoroughly washing fresh produce prior to preparing or eating it.

Listeria monocytogenes: L. monocytogenes occurs widely in nature. Since the early 1900s, scientists have known that this pathogen causes infection in animals and humans. But, it wasn't until around 1980 that scientists realized that this bacterium could be conveyed by food. In fact, one of the most tragic foodborne infection outbreaks in the U.S. confirmed that food is an important source of L. monocytogenes infection.

In 1985, contaminated soft cheese was linked with 142 cases of listeriosis (the disease caused by L. monocytogenes) that resulted in 47 fatalities, including 29 infants infected during fetal life. In actuality, this organism rarely causes disease in healthy persons. However, it can be devastating for vulnerable individuals--notably those with underdeveloped immune systems (e.g., fetuses, neonates), and persons with weakened immune systems. About one-fourth of the 1600 or so Americans who develop listeriosis each year die from it.

L. monocytogenes is mostly associated with raw milk, but in most developed countries, milk is rarely the cause of listeriosis because pasteurization kills this microorganism. However, a few soft cheeses such as Brie, Camembert, and Mexican-style cheeses (e.g., Queso Blanco and Queso Fresco) are made with milk that is not pasteurized. Although soft cheeses are the primary cause of listeriosis, infections also have resulted from blue-veined cheeses, unwashed produce, and processed meats and seafood (e.g. luncheon meats, shrimp salad). L. monocytogenes also can be spread by the fecal-oral route and cross-contamination. L. monocytogenes is described as being a 'tough bug' or 'macho microbe' because it is able to survive typical cooking temperatures and the effects of food processing much better than many microorganisms. It can even continue multiplying at refrigerator temperatures. However, temperatures of 0°F (-18°C) will stop it from multiplying and temperatures above 140°F (60°C) will kill it.

Because foods associated with L. monocytogenes are not always heated before serving and because this bacterium can thrive under conditions where other bacteria have a hard time surviving, the best defense against this organism is to avoid contamination in the first place. To accomplish this in the U.S., the FDA, dairy food producers, and seafood distributors have stepped up efforts to identify potential food safety problems, recall contaminated products, and eliminate sources of contamination.

The low percentage of products found to be contaminated indicates that these efforts are paying off. An additional precautionary measure for individuals vulnerable to listeriosis is to avoid foods and food preparation techniques associated with listeriosis.

Staphylococcus aureus: S. aureus, also known as 'staph', is the most common type of bacterium that causes foodborne intoxication. As many as two in five cases of foodborne illness are caused by S. aureus toxin. The usual source of S. aureus contamination is a food handler who harbors the bacterium. S. aureus live in many people's respiratory tracts and can be transmitted to food by sneezing or coughing. These bacteria also can enter food from open cuts, sores, and pimples. It is not surprising, then, that the most 'risky' foods for staph intoxication include those that are extensively handled, such as sliced meats and salads made with chopped ingredients (e.g., potato salad or egg salad). Like most bacteria, S. aureus grow readily in protein-rich, moist foods of animal origin. Cooking will kill the bacteria, but unlike most bacterial toxins heat will not destroy the staph toxin. So, the only way to prevent staph intoxication is to prevent contamination by using safe food-handling procedures and prevent the growth of the bacteria. Bacterial growth can be prevented by thoroughly cooking food and then refrigerating it immediately.

Clostridium perfringens: C. perfringens is known as the 'café germ' or 'banquet germ' because the source of most outbreaks is food served in restaurants or events such as picnics or banquets.

The culprit food is typically a protein-rich dish in a deep pan, such as a casserole, gravy, or stew, which is made well ahead of serving, kept at temperatures in the danger zone (40 to 140E F or 5 to 60E C), and not thoroughly reheated before serving. C. perfringens thrives under these conditions because it is endospore-forming and requires at least moderately anaerobic (oxygen-free) conditions for growth. The endospores survive the initial cooking of the food, and as the temperature drops into the danger zone they germinate and grow in the food's anaerobic center. (Endospores are a dormant form certain bacteria can take that can survive stresses that would kill active bacterial cells, such as dryness and heat. When conditions favor growth, the spores become active [germinate] and bacteria multiply.)

Intoxication thus can be prevented by refrigerating foods immediately after cooking. If necessary, the food can be divided into shallow pans so that it chills rapidly. The toxin produced by C. perfringens can be inactivated by heat (unlike staph toxin), so thoroughly reheating a food before serving will prevent intoxication. C. perfringens is ubiquitous, occurring naturally in soil, water, dust, and sewage--it can contaminate food when any of these come in contact with food. It also can be spread by cross-contamination from one food to another.

Clostridium botulinum: The toxin produced by C. botulinum, called botulin, is the single most deadly poison known. An amount equal in size to a grain of salt can kill several people in less than an hour. Ten pounds could kill everyone on earth. It is fortunate that this type of foodborne intoxication, known as botulism, is rare because two out of three cases result in death.

Like its relative C. perfringens, C. botulinum is an endospore-forming anaerobe that is ubiquitously present in soil and probably contaminates virtually all foods. This bacterium is fairly sensitive to acid conditions and generally will not grow in acid food, but it can germinate, grow, and produce its deadly toxin in any non-acid, moderately anaerobic food. That is why the classic source of botulin is canned or bottled non-acid foods, such as mushrooms, corn, peas, and meats that have been incorrectly processed.

Correct processing of such foods involves heating them to a temperature that will destroy the C. botulinum endospores as well as the bacteria and toxin. Virtually all commercially canned and bottled foods have been correctly processed and are safe. Home-canned non-acid foods may be risky. A few cases of botulism have been associated with the kinds of foods that typically cause C. perfringens outbreaks—that is, foods with anaerobic centers such as macaroni salad, casseroles, and stew. Smoked fish have been a culprit, too.

It is important to know that honey poses a botulism risk to infants, although not to adults. Honey contains C. botulinum endospores, and these spores can germinate and multiply in the gastrointestinal tracts of infants less than one year old. Infants should never be fed honey. The botulin toxin injures the body by irreversibly attaching itself to nerve endings and blocking nerve impulses thereby causing muscle weakness and paralysis. Botulin tends to start with the cranial nerves and then work its way symmetrically down the body. When the cranial nerves are affected the eyelids droop, the individual has difficulty swallowing, chewing, and talking, and experiences dizziness and double vision---victims often are mistakenly thought to be inebriated. As the toxin moves downward, the arms and legs become paralyzed. Once the toxin attaches itself to the nerves that control the muscles in the chest and diaphragm, respiration is inhibited and the victim dies of asphyxiation. Victims are treated with an antitoxin that destroys the botulin toxin that has not yet attached itself to nerve endings. Unfortunately, the antitoxin has no effect on the toxin that is already attached to nerve endings. So, the key to recovery is a quick diagnosis and immediate administration of antitoxin.

The longer it takes to administer the antitoxin, the more nerve endings will be damaged by the toxin and the greater the recovery time will be. Respiratory support is essential if the nerves that control the muscles in the chest and diaphragm have been affected by the toxin. Generally, recovery is a slow process because damaged nerves take months or even years to fully regenerate. The biggest problem with getting a quick diagnosis is that botulism is so rare that many physicians have never seen a case. By the time the correct diagnosis is made and the antitoxin is administered, significant nerve damage, or even death, may have occurred. Thus, prevention is the only good way to deal with this disease.

Botulism can be prevented by checking food cans and jars closely and discarding any that leak, bulge, have holes, are rusted, or contain food that looks or smells odd or spurts out when the container is opened. If food is suspected of containing the botulin, don't take any chances--discard the food so that no person or animal can eat it. Tasting just one corn kernel contaminated with botulin can be fatal. Also, avoid smelling or touching the food because the toxin also can enter the body through the lungs or a cut in the skin. When serving low-acid home canned foods (e.g., meats and most vegetables), many food scientists recommend that these foods be boiled for 15 minutes before they are tasted because heat will destroy any C. botulinum and botulin toxin they might contain.

Yersinia enterocolitica: Y. enterocolitica is a relatively rare cause of foodborne infection, but the resulting disease can be severe and linger for a year or longer. Victims may experience abdominal pain so severe that it mimics appendicitis. In fact, this bacterium has caused several individuals to undergo unnecessary appendectomies. The foods most frequently implicated as the source of Y. enterocolitica are undercooked meats, raw milk, and foods prepared with contaminated water. This bacterium multiplies slowly at refrigerator temperatures, but thorough cooking and pasteurization destroy it and prevent infection.

Vibrio: Vibrio cholerae causes the deadly foodborne infection cholera, a disease characterized by relentless diarrhea and often by vomiting. Cholera, a major public health problem in developing countries, is spread by the feces of infected individuals. Raw shellfish are the primary food source of this illness. With medical treatment, victims recover in a few days, however without treatment, more than 60 percent die. Death results from dehydration caused by diarrhea, which leads to circulatory collapse. Safe food-handling procedures and improved sewage treatment methods can prevent cholera. Cholera currently causes epidemics only in countries where sanitation is poor. A cholera epidemic raged throughout South America in the early 1990s infecting more than a million people and killing over 5,000.

Two other Vibrio species that cause foodborne disease are associated mainly with inadequately cooked shellfish, particularly oysters and shrimp. Vibrio vulnificus is found in warm seawaters and causes only about 100 illnesses in the U.S. each year, but 40 to 65 percent of the victims die. Vibrio parahaemolyticus is the main cause of foodborne illness in Japan; very few cases have been identified in the U.S.

Shigella: Shigella shares many similarities with V. cholerae. That is, it too is spread by the feces of infected individuals, is most common in areas with inadequate sanitation, and can be prevented by safe food-handling procedures and improved sewage treatment. And like cholera, death from Shigella infection results from dehydration caused by diarrhea.

Viral Foodborne Illnesses

Viruses, like bacteria, are widely dispersed in nature and injure the body directly or by making a toxin. Several viruses, such as hepatitis A virus, Norwalk virus, and rotaviruses, are known to cause foodborne infections. These viruses are spread just as bacteria are: by the fecal-oral route, cross-contamination, and infected food handlers. Unlike bacteria, viruses can reproduce only after invading the body's cells. Thus, the key to preventing foodborne viral illnesses is to use sanitary food preparation practices to keep viruses from contaminating food and to cook food thoroughly to kill any that found their way into food.

Hepatitis A: Hepatitis A is a contagious liver infection that can be a very serious, sometimes fatal illness that may be food or waterborne. Hepatitis A attacks the liver causing jaundice, very yellow urine, and liver damage. In industrialized countries, the number of reported cases ranges from about 10 to 50 per 100,000 people each year. It is one of the most commonly reported infectious diseases in the U.S. In developing and Eastern European countries, 50 to 300 cases per 100,000 people are reported annually. Although the overall incidence of this illness is low, it is particularly common among those who live in crowded quarters, lack running water, and have poor sanitation. For instance, researchers reported that individuals living in some poverty stricken areas are so susceptible to hepatitis A infection that more than 80 percent of the adults and a third of the children have suffered from this illness.

Undercooked shellfish harvested from sewage contaminated waterways and inadequately washed produce are the most common sources of hepatitis A. Consuming contaminated water or ice also can lead to this viral infection. This virus can survive for a long time at room temperature and is not affected by freezing. Heat destroys the hepatitis A virus, so this disease can be avoided by cooking foods thoroughly. Safe food-handling procedures will minimize its spread via infected food handlers. Chlorination of water supplies also kills this virus and halts its spread.

A vaccination also is available to prevent hepatitis A. Universal immunization is highly recommended because vaccination could successfully control hepatitis A. However, currently vaccine cost and availability preclude such a recommendation. Nonetheless, those at high risk of this disease should get a hepatitis A vaccine. Persons who should get the hepatitis A vaccine include anyone age 2 and over who will be traveling or working in countries with high rates of this disease, particularly Central and South America, the Caribbean, Mexico, Africa, southern or eastern Europe, and Asia (except Japan). Others who should get this vaccine are those living in communities with prolonged outbreaks or high rates of hepatitis A, homosexual men, those who use intravenous street drugs, chronic liver disease patients, and people receiving blood clotting factor concentrates such as hemophilia patients.

Rotaviruses: Although anyone at any age is susceptible to rotavirus infection, this infection is particularly common in children. In fact, experts believe that nearly every child on earth will experience a rotavirus infection at least once before they reach age five. Each year in the U.S., severe rotavirus infections cause thousands of children between the ages of 3 and 35 months to be hospitalized or need emergency room treatment. Foods are usually contaminated with rotaviruses by infected food handlers and sewage contaminated water. Safe food-handling procedures will minimize its spread via infected food handlers. Although a vaccine is available to help prevent rotavirus infections, it is not recommended for routine use in infants because of a strong association between it and bowl obstruction.

Norwalk Viruses : In the U.S., only the common cold is more frequent than viral gastroenteritis—fully one-third of the cases among those over the age of two are attributed to Norwalk viruses. This virus was first identified after an outbreak of gastrointestinal disease in Norwalk, Ohio in 1972. Since that incident, other similar viruses have been identified and are sometimes termed 'Norwalk-like viruses'. In developing countries, Norwalk viruses are so common that a very high percentage of children develop immunity at an early age. In the U.S., the percentage having immunity rises with age, reaching approximately half the population by age 18. Unfortunately, immunity is not permanent and re-infection can occur. But, generally the illness that results from Norwalk viruses is mild and brief. Foods are contaminated with Norwalk viruses via the fecal-oral route and contaminated water. Salads, insufficiently cooked clams and oysters, ice, and water are the most commonly implicated foods. Safe food handling procedures, thorough washing of fresh produce with clean water, thorough cooking of shellfish, and sanitary disposal of sewage helps to prevent this disease.

Molds

Molds are a type of fungus that spread from place to place through the air like dandelion seeds. They grow best in humid, dark places where air circulates. When conditions are right, the mold grows by sending root-like 'threads' deep into the food it lives on and forming endospores on the outside of food. These endospores give mold the fuzzy, colorful look you see and are the form in which the mold travels to new locations. The foods most likely to mold in U.S. homes are cheese, breads, and fresh produce.

Thousands of types of molds grow on foods: Most just alter the color, texture, taste, and/or odor of foods, making them unpalatable and inedible. Some destroy crops and shorten storage times. Others cause allergies or respiratory problems. A few fungi produce toxins known as mycotoxins ('myco' is the prefix meaning 'mold') which cause blood diseases, nervous system disorders, and kidney and liver damage. The most important mycotoxins are aflatoxin, ergot, and those produced by the Fusaria fungi. Aflatoxin is produced by a mold that attacks peanuts, tree nuts, corn, and oilseeds and is a known carcinogen. Ergot is produced by a dark purple mold that grows on improperly stored grains, especially rye. It is a natural source of lysergic acid diethylamide (LSD) and is a powerful hallucinogen. Ergot poisoning can cause spontaneous abortion and constrict blood flow to the arms and legs so severely that gangrene develops. Several types of Fusaria fungi can grow on grains stored for long periods, and produce deadly mycotoxins.

Mycotoxins are rarely a problem in most industrial nations because food production practices are designed to minimize mold growth. In addition, food producers and government inspectors closely monitor foods to detect molds and destroy any foods found to contain them. Unfortunately, mycotoxin poisonings are frequent in other parts of the world. For example, in India in 1975 an outbreak of aflatoxin poisoning caused liver damage in many people and killed some. Mycotoxins, from Fusaria involving mainly millet and other cereal grains stored for long periods, are a public health problem in the countries that once formed the Soviet Union.

To prevent molds from invading food, keep foods covered to prevent them from becoming home to airborne mold endospores. Another way to prevent the spread of mold is to scrub mold off refrigerator walls and door seals. Also, launder dish cloths and sponges often; a musty smell means they are spreading mold. It also is important to inspect foods carefully for signs of mold growth when grocery shopping and just before preparing them. Yet another prevention method is to eat foods as soon after purchasing as possible—the longer they are stored, the more likely they are to mold.

Despite all precautions, mold still invades many foods. Food covered with mold should be wrapped and thrown away so that no person or animal can eat it. Avoid sniffing the food because mold spores can enter the lungs and cause respiratory difficulties. Next, clean the area where the moldy food was sitting and check nearby foods for mold (mold spreads fast, especially in fruits and vegetables). If a piece of food has only a small spot of mold and is of a firm type (e.g., hard cheeses, carrots, cabbage, potatoes) part of the food may be salvaged by carving away at least an inch around and below the moldy area. Foods that are soft or liquid (e.g., lettuce, tomatoes, jam, cottage cheese, syrup, juice) should be discarded even if they only have a trace of mold. Don't try to salvage moldy bread, baked goods, flour, grains, legumes, nuts, and peanut butter; they may contain harmful toxins.

Parasitic Foodborne Illnesses

Parasites live in or on another organism, known as the host, from which they absorb nutrients. Humans may serve as the host to parasites. These tiny ravagers rob millions of people around the globe of their health and, in some cases, their lives. Those hardest hit live in tropical countries where poor sanitation fosters the growth of parasites. However, epidemiologists report that parasitic infections seem to be on the increase in the U.S. and other industrialized countries. Parasitic infections may be transmitted in many ways, including contaminated foods.

The more than 80 foodborne parasites known to affect humans include mainly two types: helminths (worms) and protozoa (one-celled animals). The most common foodborne helminths in the U.S. are tapeworms, Trichinella spiralis, and anisakids.

Tapeworms: These long, flat worms have heads equipped with suckers and hooks that lock the worms onto the host's intestinal tract. Tapeworm cysts or 'eggs' are found in raw and undercooked beef, fish, and pork. Within a few days of being eaten, the tapeworm cysts germinate and the worms begin growing. Most who have tapeworms don't realize it until they excrete tapeworm segments or a living tapeworm in their feces. In cases where the tapeworms grow excessively long (i.e., several yards), they may cause intestinal blockage and steal enough nutrients from their host to cause nutrient deficiencies. Tapeworms are easy to avoid because thorough cooking kills the cysts. A cyst is a structure formed by certain microorganisms that encases them, puts them in a dormant state, and enables them to survive harsh environmental conditions.

Trichinella spiralis: This parasite infects some pigs and wild game. Humans may develop the disease trichinosis if they eat undercooked pork or game meat containing the larvae of this parasitic roundworm. Ingested larvae mature and reproduce in the human intestinal tract, and then they die and leave the body in the feces. Their larvae, however, are left behind. The larvae may bore through the intestinal tract and travel via the blood or lymph vessels to muscles where they embed themselves, mature, and live. The severity of trichinosis symptoms depends on the number of larvae consumed. People who eat a few larvae usually don't know it, but if they eat a large amount, they will often experience intestinal upset, sore muscles, and difficulty talking, swallowing and breathing. The problem with trichinosis is that once symptoms develop, a great deal of damage has already been done to the muscles. Fortunately, there are less than 100 cases of trichinosis in the U.S. yearly mainly because most people know that pork must be cooked thoroughly and because legislation now requires that any garbage fed to pigs must be cooked, which kills any larvae.

Trichinosis may be on the down swing in the U.S., but fish-borne parasitic illnesses, such as anisakiasis, are on rise. This increase corresponds to the growing popularity of raw fish dishes, like sushi, sashimi, ceviche, and gravlax. Anisakiasis is caused by the larvae of anisakids worms boring into the stomach or intestinal lining. Usually these roundworms die or do not stay long because humans are not their usual host. They may be coughed or vomited up. Some infected individuals may pull this spaghetti-shaped worn out of their throats after feel a tickling at the back of their throats. In some cases, anisakiasis causes severe stomach pain that persists until the larvae are removed surgically. To help prevent parasite ridden fish from reaching consumers, fish processors thoroughly inspect species that are likely to carry parasites. However, to be completely safe, it is important to thoroughly cook fish or freeze it at 0°F (-18°C) for 72 hours or more before preparing it.

Toxoplasma gondii. Another common parasitic disease, toxoplasmosis, is caused by a protozoan parasite known as Toxoplasma gondii. When this parasite infects a human or other animal, it enters their tissues where it forms parasite-filled cysts. These cysts typically cause few or no symptoms in healthy adults unless they are numerous or happen to be located in a sensitive place such as the brain. However, toxoplasmosis is very dangerous for immuno-suppressed individuals and fetuses of pregnant women. T. gondii parasites frequently infect cats and then are excreted in cat feces, so litter boxes are a common source of human infection. The infection also can be caused by eating undercooked meat from infected animals or by eating vegetables grown in soil contaminated with infectious feces, typically cat feces. Infection may be avoided by cooking meat thoroughly, washing vegetables well, and washing hands carefully after cleaning a cat's litter box. Pregnant women should be particularly careful to avoid all contact with cat feces and never clean litter boxes.

Giardia lamblia and Cryptosporidium parvum: These two protozoan parasites are becoming all too common in the U.S. G. lamblia is frequently spread via the fecal-oral route and is a fairly common problem in day care centers. Water contaminated with C. parvum cysts from the fecal matter of mammals and foods prepared with this water have caused several major outbreaks in the U.S. in recent years. When the presence of these and other protozoan parasites is detected in municipal water supplies, households are usually instructed to boil their tap water or use bottled water until the water supply is declared safe. It may take weeks to lower the numbers of these parasites to a level that isn't likely to cause disease because these parasites are so small they may slip past the water filters municipal water companies commonly used. Also, these parasites may be able to withstand chlorine treatments used to sanitize water supplies.

Keeping Food Safe to Eat

Although government agencies have an official responsibility to ensure the safety of the food supply, every person who handles food, including food producers, processors, shippers, foods store workers, and consumers, also assume some of this responsibility. Moreover, the government has no authority in one place where many foodborne illnesses start--the home kitchen. Most home kitchens would flunk a sanitation inspection! In one study, 99 percent of the households failed a kitchen inspection test based on guidelines adapted from the

National Restaurant Association. Even worse is that participants in this study knew someone would be visiting their home to observe and evaluate their kitchen practices—even with advance preparation, less than one percent met the minimum criteria for acceptable performance. The Centers for Disease Control and Prevention estimate that 85 percent of all foodborne illness could be avoided if people took precautionary steps in their own homes.

To help educators focus their efforts on the most critical food handling behaviors, the WHO developed Golden Rules for Safe Food Preparation (click to enlarge). In the U.S., government and private sector agencies formed the Partnership for Food Safety Education which launched the Fight BAC! campaign in 1997 to teach consumers about safe food handling. In addition, numerous educational materials are available. The basic steps consumers can take to protect themselves against pathogens, especially bacterial pathogens, and to otherwise ensure the food they eat at home is safe and contains as few pathogens as possible, are described below.

Practice Good Personal Hygiene: Pathogenic microorganisms found on skin, hair, and clothes can get into food and cause foodborne illness. Here's what consumers can do to avoid contaminating food during preparation.

Wash their hands with hot, soapy water before handling foods and during food preparation right after coughing, sneezing, going to the bathroom, eating, drinking, touching bare parts of their bodies, or handling raw animal flesh, unwashed produce, or dirty dishes or food preparation equipment.

— Wear clean clothes and tie back long hair.

— Avoid preparing food when sick.

— Cover wounds, burns, sores, and infected areas while preparing food.

Keep the Kitchen Clean: Pathogenic microorganisms thrive in damp, dirty areas of the kitchen like cracks and dark corners.

Pests, such as insects and mice, like dirty kitchens, too. They move in when crumbs, food spills, and garbage are left in the kitchen and spread microorganisms as they climb over counters, dishes, and food. Here's how to keep harmful microorganisms and pests under control.

— Wash all work surfaces (e.g., countertops, cutting boards) with soap and water and rinse well before using them and after they come in contact with raw animal flesh, eggs, or unwashed produce to avoid cross-contamination.

— Wash dish towels and sponges often because they teem with bacteria which easily spread to and from the hands and around the kitchen as towels or sponges are used.

— Sweep the floor regularly, wipe up spills as soon as they happen, and keep the garbage can covered. Pests like crumbs, spills, and garbage. And, bacteria grow quickly in spills.

Handle Foods Safely: Careless food handling sets the stage for bacterial growth and cross contamination. Here's how to handle foods safely.

— Wash raw fruits and vegetables thoroughly to remove soil particles and microorganisms. Some people may want to peel them and throw away outer leaves of cabbage and lettuce.

— Keep raw foods, especially animal flesh and its juices, separated from cooked foods or foods that won't be cooked.

— Keep dirty utensils and dishes separated from clean dishes and food.

— Use a clean spoon each time food is tasted during preparation.

— Handle foods as little as possible; even clean hands carry small amounts of harmful pathogens.

— Take groceries home right after shopping and put frozen

and refrigerated foods away immediately. Avoid storing canned and dry foods under a sink or near a range because bacteria and molds thrive in moist, warm places.

Follow the storage and preparation directions on food packages.

— Use food as soon after purchasing it as possible. Clean out the refrigerator, freezer, and pantry often, discarding spoiled foods or those in torn or damaged containers; microorganisms and pests may have gotten into them.

— Keep foods out of the danger zone. Bacteria grow fastest at danger zone temperatures (i.e., 40 to 140°F or 5 to 60° C). Here's how to curtail bacterial proliferation and foodborne illness.

— Keep refrigerator temperatures between 32 and 40°F (0-4°C) and freezer temperatures at 0°F or (-18°C) or below. Leave cold foods in the refrigerator or freezer until they are needed. It is not safe to bring animal flesh, eggs, milk, and other protein-rich foods to room temperature before cooking them.

— Thaw frozen foods of animal origin in a microwave oven, in a refrigerator, or under cold running water. Thawing food on the countertop gives bacteria a chance to multiply. Once thawed, refrigerate or cook immediately.

Thoroughly cook animal flesh. Between 25 and 75 percent of the meat sold is retail outlets may be contaminated with at least one pathogen, but most microorganisms are killed when meat and fish reach 160°F (71°C) and poultry reaches 180°F the (82°C). Common visual cues that consumers use to determine doneness may not ensure safety. Thus, a thermometer should be used to be sure they are cooked to safe temperatures. In the U.S., the Food Safety Inspection Service has launched an educational campaign called "Thermy" to encourage consumer to use thermometers.

Keep cooked foods at 140°F (60°C) or higher until they are served. Do not allow them to remain at danger zone temperatures for more than 2 hours. Store leftovers right away. Keep leftovers no more than 3 days and reheat them to at least 165°F (74°C) to destroy microorganisms that contaminated the food after it was cooked.

Pack lunches and picnics in an insulated cooler. Put the cooler in a cool location, out of direct sunlight. Avoid recipes in which eggs remain raw or only partly cooked (e.g., eggnog, mousse) or use only pasteurized eggs in these recipes. Eggs are safe to eat when the yolk and white are firm; Salmonella bacteria may still survive in eggs cooked 'sunny side up' or soft-scrambled.

Avoid foods from unsafe sources. Some foods pose greater food safety hazards than others. For example, fresh sprouts often are contaminated with harmful bacteria and because they are fragile and eaten raw, it is difficult to reduce the amount of bacteria they contain.

— Avoid eating raw sprouts.

— Only drink pasteurized milk and juices.

— Avoid eating raw or undercooked meat, fish, shellfish, poultry, and eggs.

— If at increased risk for foodborne illness, avoid soft cheeses, cold deli salads, and cold smoked fish and heat hot dogs and deli meats to 165°F (75° C) before consumption.

When shopping, reject cans that are damaged, jars that aren't tightly closed, and frozen foods that are soft, soggy, or have stained packages. These signs indicate that the food inside the package may be unsafe to eat. Check the dates on foods and never buy outdated foods.

Knowing that the food on the dinner table could make someone sick is a disturbing thought. But, even worse is knowing that the incidence of foodborne illness could be greatly reduced by taking a few simple precautions. Yet, few health education classes address this topic. As we enter the 21st century, it is vital to recognized that all health professionals play critical roles in decreasing the burden of foodborne illness.

Nutritional Problems

Kidney Diseases

Nutrition may affect persons who have, or are at risk for developing renal disease. The intake of certain nutrients may influence the rate of progression of renal failure in persons with underlying renal disease. High-protein diets can strain the kidneys to the point of failure. This is substantiated by the findings that the prevalence of stone disease in vegetarians is only about 50% of that in the general population. A high intake of animal protein increases the urinary excretion of calcium and oxalate and the accompanying increase in purine intake increases uric acid excretion. Functioning kidneys regulate the composition and volume of body fluids within very narrow limits. They do so by balancing intake and excretion of body fluids and waste products derived from metabolic processes. If the kidneys fail to maintain homeostasis, a wide range of potentially lethal metabolic disorders can develop throughout the body.

The kidneys remove unwanted salts, waste products, and other chemicals from the plasma along with the water in which they are dissolved. When the concentration of certain salts in urine exceeds the limits of solubility, the salts crystallize and form stones within the kidneys. Treatment of these conditions by diet or drugs is aimed at reducing the concentration of stone-forming substances in the urine. The principal means to this end is to increase urine production by drinking water throughout the day unless on a low-fluid regimen. The substances found most frequently in kidney stones include calcium, oxalate, phosphate, uric acid, and cystine. Usually these substances are derived from foods, but oxalate and uric acid can also be synthesized endogenously.

Dietary measures to reduce oxalate include restriction of oxalate-rich foods, such as beetroot, rhubarb, spinach, chocolate, and tea, and restriction of excessive intake of ascorbic acid, which is metabolized to oxalate. Uric acid stones are treated with diets low in purine-rich foods, such as organ meats, fish, shellfish, and legumes.

Persons with cystine-containing stones respond successfully to low protein diets. Calcium phosphate stones are treated successfully with high-phosphate diets that increase urinary excretion of pyrophosphate, an inhibitor of calcium crystallization. Chronic renal failure is the consequence of longstanding and progressive renal damage and is usually irreversible. Chronicrenal failure causes extensive disorders in appetite as well as in the body's absorption, excretion, and metabolism of many nutrients. Consequently, nutritional therapy is essential in managing this condition.

The chronic renal failure patient is also likely to accumulate certain potentially toxic chemicals that normally are ingested in small amounts and excreted in the urine. Aluminum is such a toxin; it can cause severe bone disease, dementia, muscle weakness, and anaemia in persons with kidney failure. Treatment of renal disease may demand severe dietary restrictions or induce nutrient losses. Dietary management of this condition, therefore, must provide protein, energy, and other essential nutrients in amounts adequate to avoid deficiencies but sufficiently restricted to avoid stressing the diminished excretory capacity of the diseased kidney.

The goals of nutritional therapy for both acute and chronic renal failure are to maintain optimal nutritional status, to minimize the toxic effects of excess urea in the blood, to prevent loss of lean body mass, to promote patient well-being, to retard the progression of renal failure, and to postpone initiation of dialysis. These goals are accomplished with the following methods:-

— *Restricting fluid intake:* Energy, protein, and other essential nutrients are provided in as small a fluid volume as is possible to maintain water balance.

— *Restricting protein:* Nitrogen balance must be maintained without any unnecessary accumulation of urea or other toxic nitrogenous waste products. To enhance incorporation of amino acids into body protein and to reduce protein breakdown in more severely ill persons, dietary protein or supplements of high biologic value (containing a high proportion of essential amino acids) are often recommended.

— *Increasing energy intake:* The higher the energy intake, the less dietary protein is required to maintain nitrogen balance. Increasing the carbohydrate and fat content of the diet provides calories that do not stress the compromised excretory capacity of the kidney. Patients with acute renal failure, however, are often unable to tolerate high carbohydrate loads and may require insulin administration.

Regulating Phosphate, Calcium, and Magnesium Intake

Phosphate restriction is necessary to prevent the metabolic bone disease that often accompanies renal failure, phosphate levels can be regulated with phosphate-binding agents that cause dietary phosphate to be excreted rather than absorbed. Calcium may be administered as a supplement as needed. Excessive magnesium levels are not usually present unless magnesium-containing antacids are used, avoiding them or using magnesium-binding agents prevents toxic accumulation of this substance.

Supplementing vitamins and trace elements: Supplemental water-soluble vitamins and trace elements are usually used to compensate for inadequate intake and losses in dialysis.

Providing appropriate counselling and support: Diets for renal patients are based on contradictory principles (meet nutritional needs but restrict protein and phosphorus), are especially restrictive, and require careful monitoring of the patient's nutritional status. Thus, trained nutrition professionals are usually essential for dietary management.

Gastrointestinal Diseases

The gastrointestinal system extracts essential vitamins and minerals from diverse plant and animal foods and breaks down the carbohydrate, protein, and fat molecules to smaller subunits that can be absorbed. It accomplishes these tasks by means of the various digestive organs of the body and the enzymes. The diet must provide, sufficient nutrients and energy to synthesize the rapidly renewing cells that line the gastrointestinal tract, the enzymes that digest and transport nutrients across the intestinal walls, and other hormones that control these processes. Digestive function can be seriously disrupted by inadequate nutrition.

Diseases of the gastrointestinal tract will unavoidably have profound effects on nutritional and metabolic processes. Loss of body weight is often an indication of gastrointestinal disease and a diet history may reveal obvious nutritional deficiencies associated with the underlying disease, eating problems, and psychological problems. Dietary fat, fiber, and alcohol are significant factors associated with gastrointestinal diseases. Higher intakes of dietary fiber can prevent or relieve symptoms of constipation and chronic diverticular disease. Individuals with celiac disease should obtain information on foods free of wheat gluten. Those with inflammatory bowel disease, heart-burn, and ulcers should follow diets appropriate to their conditions.

Diseases of the Mouth

Dental caries result from demineralization of the enamel surface of the tooth by acids produced from sugars. Initially mineral disappears from the sub-surface of the tooth and if this process is not addressed a cavity will develop in which more bacterial growth can occur causing further dissolution of enamel. Eventually the tooth may be lost. The presence in the mouth of fermentable sugars is essential for the development of dental caries. Within minutes of consumption sugars cause the pH in dental plaque to fall below the critical pH for enamel dissolution. This fall in pH will occur irrespective of the amount of sugar consumed or whether it comes from fruit or chocolate.

The normal oral pH of 7.0 will only be restored about 30 minutes after the sugar has finally been swallowed. Normally the pH will return sooner if the item is consumed quickly rather than if eaten slowly over a long period of time. Acidic foods, such as citrus fruits and cola drinks, lower the mouth pH and hence produce cariogenic conditions. Finishing a meal with an alkaline food, such as cheese, milk, or peanuts can help to raise the pH of the mouth.

Fluoride can increase enamel resistance by the formation of fluorhydroxyapatite crystals in the tooth which are more resistant to acid erosion. The maximum benefit from fluoride is obtained if it is available during tooth formation. Once the tooth has emerged, further protection can be obtained from topical or dietary fluoride. Deficiency of certain vitamins may produce inflammation of the gums and the teeth may become loose from the lack of cement which normally holds them to the jaw. A lack of vitamin C causes scurvy, a weakening of periodontal fibers and the teeth may become loose and fall out. The gums become tender and bleed easily. Treatment is by vitamin therapy and sources of vitamin C should be included in the diet regularly.

Deficiency of vitamin D causes defective calcification of the dentine of the teeth and may increase susceptibility to dental caries. Eruption of the teeth may be delayed in children with rickets. Vitamin D therapy should be given and good sources of vitamin D taken in the diet, together with exposure to sunlight where possible.

Disorders of the Oesophagus

The diaphragm has several openings through which the abdominal viscera can enter the thorax. The opening for the oesophagus, the hiatus, is loosely attached to the oesophagus. In middle age this attachment weakens and in overweight people additional abdominal weight puts extra strain on the hiatus which herniates. A low fiber diet which results in constipation causes straining when the bowels are opened and weakening of the hiatus. The major symptoms of hiatus hernia are those of reflux and oesophagitis and the sensation of food 'sticking'. The refluxed contents of the stomach may contain partly digested foods, acids and enzymes. It is possibly this combination which causes mucosal damage and oesophagitis. Symptoms develop if reflux becomes frequent and the mucosa of the oesophagus becomes sensitive to the acidic reflux. Fatty foods, chocolate, coffee, alcohol, spicy foods and citrus juices lower sphincter pressure and may induce reflux.

Cystic Fibrosis

Cystic fibrosis (CF) is a generalized hereditary condition characterized by chronic pulmonary disease, reduced secretion of water and bicarbonate, pancreatic enzyme deficiency and abnormally high concentrations of electrolytes in the sweat. Progressive malnutrition and poor growth are common features of CF and need to be addressed by diet therapy. It is important to provide the CF patient with the optimum diet for the potential for growth to be fulfilled and resistance to infection maximized.

Energy intake is generally increased by 50% more than the Recommended Daily Requirement. In order to achieve an adequate energy intake, effective use should be made of suitable energysupplements such as glucose polymers and glucose drinks. Fat intake should be normal and frequent snacks should be encouraged. Deficiencies of vitamins A, D, E and K are well documented. Daily supplementation of 8000 IU of vitamin A, 20 μg of vitamin D, and 200 mg of vitamin E is currently advised. Deficiency of vitamin K has been noted in patients with liver disease and in young infants with CF. A supplementation is only necessary if deficiency has been demonstrated.

Lactose Intolerance

Lactose (milk sugar) is digested in the small intestine by the enzyme lactase. An insufficiency of lactase, in the small intestine, results in undigested lactose to pass into the large intestine where it is fermented by bacteria with the production of lactic acid. This accumulation of lactic acid is characterized by abdominal discomfort, pain, and diarrhea, the condition known as lactose intolerance. After the age of 5 the genetic absence of lactase occurs among remarkably high proportions of Asians (95 percent), Africans (99 percent), American Indians (95 percent), and black Americans (75 percent), as well as among a significant proportion of healthy Caucasians.

The origin of racial lactose intolerance is not entirely clear. It may be a genetic difference or it may be that the custom of drinking milk, which is common among Caucasians, results in the continued production of lactase. Many other races do not take much milk after infancy, so the enzyme diminishes or disappears completely. For practical purposes, no differentiation is usually made between cows milk and goats or sheeps milk. For people who are milk intolerant a wide range of soya based foods are available.

Infections and Immunity

The immune system protects the body against infection by producing specific substances in response to foreign materials called antigens. Immunity to specific antigens occurs through the cooperative interactions of two subsets of blood cells, T lymphocytes and B lymphocytes. There are several subtypes of T lymphocytes, each with specific functions. Helper and suppressor T lymphocytes regulate the quantities of antibodies produced, while killer T lymphocytes respond selectively to foreign material, search and destroy internally infected, or malignant body cells. Severe infections can compromise nutritional status through a variety of mechanisms: hypermetabolism, appetite depression, decreased absorption of nutrients, altered nutrient metabolism, increased nutrient excretion, and internal diversion of nutrients. additional nutrient losses occur with vomiting, diarrhea, and sweating.

Hypermetabolism

Fever causes metabolic rates to increase. This hypermetabolism affects all cells in the body. Because this extra energy comes largely from amino acid metabolism the body stores of muscle protein amino acids are rapidly depleted. Loss of nutrients also occur during sweating associated with fever. Controlling the infection reduces fever and losses of body nutrients. Severe loss of appetite is a common symptom during most infectious diseases and often leads to an almost total cessation of food consumption. Vomiting and diarrhea further reduce the absorption of nutrients. Antibiotics and other medications also modify intestinal absorption. Excess nitrogen is metabolized to urea and excreted in the urine. Even brief viral infections and brief fevers induced by bacterial infections can cause sizable losses of nitrogen.

Tissue and plasma concentrations of most vitamins decline during infections, because of increased metabolism or excretion. The accelerated metabolism or loss of vitamins during infections may precipitate recognizable deficiency states.

Food Associated Illnesses

Adverse reactions to food involve immunologic and nonimmunologic mechanisms. Immunologic reactions are known as food allergies. Nonimmunologic intolerances include those that are biochemical or psychologic. Food allergies are examples of the negative consequences of immune function on the gastrointestinal tract, skin, lungs, and other organs. The most common foods to which people are allergic are eggs, milk, fish, shellfish, chicken, wheat, and nuts. Symptoms include acute abdominal pain, swelling, nausea,vomiting, rashes, chronic itching, headache, tension, and fatigue. The causes of nonimmunologic adverse reactions to foods include food toxicities, food poisonings, and pharmacologic or metabolic reactions. Such intolerances occur more frequently than true food allergies and are related to dose as well as to the concurrent presence of medications, other diseases, or genetic errors of metabolism.

Sulfites

Approximately 10 percent of peopl with asthma are sensitive to ingestion of sulphite, which induces asthma. Foods containing sulfur dioxide, as a preservative, should be used with caution. FDA has taken two major steps to protect consumers who are sensitive to sulfites in food. No longer can these preservatives be used on raw fruits and vegetables. And processed foods that contain sulfites will have to say so on the package label.

The allergic-type reactions range from mild to severe, and in some cases can cause death. "Sulfites" or "sulfating agents" are general terms used to describe sulfur based substances that have been in widespread use for many years by the food and drug industries. They include sulfur dioxide, sodium sulfite, sodium and potassium bisulfite, and sodium and potassium metabisulfite. Although they have various permitted uses, their primary function is as a preservative or antioxidant to prevent or reduce spoilage and discolouration during the preparation, storage and distribution of many foods. There is some evidence that some non-asthmatics also can suffer adverse reactions to sulfites. For example, out of more than 500 reports of sulfite reactions investigated by the FDA, about one-fourth involved people who had no known history of asthma.

Asthma is also induced by tartrazine, a yellow dye used to color medicines, soft drinks, and foods. Tartrazine can also cause hyperactivity in sensitive individuals. It has no nutritional value. Because of the negative effects associated with tartrazine, foods and drinks containing it should be avoided. Other substances that cause adverse reaction or neurologic disorders are monosodium glutamate (MSG) and the preservative benzoic acid. Psychologic mechanisms can provoke physical and mental symptoms of food sensitivity that do not appear to be medicated by the immune system. In individuals with psychologically induced allergic symptoms no physiologic or biochemical nonimmunologic mechanisms can be identified. Individuals with food intolerances should exclude the offending foods from their diet. Those with potentially life-threatening sensitivities should carry an epinephrine-containing syringe and wear a bracelet identifying the problem.

HIV Infection and AIDS

Acquired immunodeficiency syndrome (AIDS), caused by the human immunodeficiency virus (HIV), is a disease with multiple pathologies, most of which are the consequence of a profound immunodeficiency. Weight loss and deteriorating nutritional status are critical features of the AIDS disease. Anorexia, nausea and vomiting, fever, and diarrhea are common features of advanced AIDS, as are malabsorption of fats, carbohydrates, and protein. Immune abnormalities resulting from malnutrition seen in AIDS implies that malnutrition might predispose to AIDS or that nutritional therapy might improve immune status and prevent AIDS.

Anemia

Anaemia occurs when the concentration of the pigment haemoglobin in red blood cells falls below normal. Haemoglobin is essential for delivering oxygen from the lungs to the body tissues. Iron was one of the first substances identified as essential in the human diet. The physiologic function of iron in haemoglobin and its role in anaemia was determined over a two hundred year period from the 1680's. Iron deficiency is the most common cause of anaemia. Anaemia signifies a blood haemoglobin concentration below the mean for normal individuals. By World Health Organization criteria, anaemia is considered to exist when the non-pregnant adult female has a haemoglobin level below 11 grams per 100 milliliter of venous blood. Although iron deficiency is generally the most common cause of anaemia, there are other nutritional, genetic, and environmental causes as well. Iron deficiency anaemia refers to anaemia that results from iron deficiency or impaired iron status. Iron dependent physiologic functions can become impaired before anaemia develops. Although iron deficiency anaemia can occur in all socioeconomic groups, it has historically been most common among the poor as is still the case today.

Causes of of Anaemia

Because the synthesis of blood cells requires many cellular and metabolic processes, a deficiency of any nutrient essential to haemoglobin production produces adverse effects on these processes. Good nutrition is fundamental to adequate red blood cell production. Nutritional anaemia may be due to a dietary deficiency of iron, folate, vitamin B12, protein, and other vitamins and minerals. Other causes of anaemia include the inherited or acquired inability to use nutrients required for haemoglobin production. Nutritional anaemia should be distinguished from deficiencies per se of iron, folate, or vitamin B12, because an individual may have manifest any one of these deficiencies without being anaemic. In iron deficiency disorders immune function and behaviour are not directly attributable to the anaemia. Similarly, the impaired nerve function of vitamin B12 deficiency occurs independently of anaemia.

Neurologic Disorders

The brain and nervous system require the full complement of essential nutrients and energy to develop and maintain their neurons and supporting cells. A deficiency of any one of these essential nutrients may impair the structure or functionality of the neurologic system. Stroke is the most common life-threatening neurologic disease. Other neurologic conditions are, epilepsy, chronic headaches, and Alzheimer's disease. The brain metabolizes 100 g to 150 g of glucose per day. During starvation, it adapts and uses ketones, derived from the breakdown of body fat stores, for energy and thus spares blood glucose and conserves body protein.

Severe deficiencies of vitamins, especially the B-complex group, impair nervous system function. Thiamin deficiency causes beriberi neuropathy as well as a peripheral neuropathy and polyneuritis that leads to paralysis of the eye muscles, loss of muscular coordination, and memory loss, especially in long-term alcoholics. Inadequate niacin intake causes pellagra, with symptoms that include intellectual impairment and dementia. Deficiency caused by vitamin B12 malabsorption in untreated pernicious anaemia, or as a result of a long term deficient vegetarian diet, can result in subacute degeneration of the spinal cord, optic nerves, cerebral white matter, and peripheral nerves.

Severely deficient intakes of other vitamins of the B-complex group also affect neurologic function. In the early stages, these symptoms are readily overcome by increased dietary intake of the appropriate vitamins, but nerve damage in later stages are irreversible. Deficiencies of other nutrients relate to defects in the nervous system function. Iodine deficiency during brain development causes mental retardation and neuromotor abnormalities. Chronic iron deficiency is associated with deficits in cognitive abilities. Vitamin E deficiency can cause spinal cord, cerebellar, and peripheral nerve degeneration with muscle wasting.

Stroke

Stroke is the sudden loss of brain function caused by thrombosis, embolism, stenosis, atherosclerosis, or haemorrhage from rupture of a cerebral artery. These events deprive the brain of oxygen and cause tissue death and irreversible damage to nervous tissue. Symptoms range from those too trivial for the victim to notice to major sensory deficits, blindness, paralysis, speech loss, coma, and death. Persons at greatest risk for stroke are those with hypertension and diabetes, and those who smoke cigarettes and display impaired cardiac function due to coronary heart disease, congestive heart failure, or hypertensive heart disease. These major risk factorsfor stroke are related to nutritional, dietary, and lifestyle factors. Moderate sodium intake, high potassium intake, vegetarian diets, calcium, weight reduction, and alcohol restriction all have been suggested as factors associated with lowering the risk factor for stroke in humans.

Headache

Headache is one of the most common complaints evaluated by neurologists. The foods most frequently implicated contain tyramines (eg. cheese, red wines), or phenylethylamine (eg. chocolates). The "Chinese Restaurant Syndrome" is associated with numbness around the mouth, tingling, flushing of the face, dizziness, and headache. This syndrome could be attributable to the high quantity of monosodium glutamate (MSG) used in the prepared foods.

Epilepsy

Low levels of magnesium can cause seizures, and the magnesium-deficient rat is used as a model of experimental epilepsy. Magnesium deficiency in humans most often results from kidney disease and is not a significant cause of epilepsy in people.

Vitamin Intake and Drug-Nutrient Interactions

Excessive intake of vitamin A causes reversible intracranial hypertension, headache, blurred vision, seizures, end encephalopathy. Excessive pyridoxine has been associated with peripheral nerve deterioration. Naturally occurring food-borne toxins also affect the mature nervous system. Specific dietary constituents, such as heavy and trace metals, may have adverse effects on the nervous systems of older adults. Increased amounts of aluminum and calcium have been reported in brains of patients with Alzheimer's disease. Some of the drugs used to treat neurologic disease can lead to vitamin deficiencies by changing the metabolism of vitamins, causing a secondary impairment of brain function. Dilantin, used to treat epilepsy, can increase folate requirements and cause vitamin K deficiency.

Hydralazine can cause neuropathy, tranquilizers such as chlorpromazine and other phenothiazines may cause hyperphagia and weight gain. Monoamine oxidase inhibitors can cause acute hypertensive crises, including excruciating headaches or fatal intracranial haemorrhages, when taken with foods or beverages high in tyramine. Caffeine, found in foods and drugs, is an active pharmacologically active agent that can enter the brain because of its lipid solubility.

Disciplines of Nutrition and Behavior

The disciplines of nutrition and behavior are not usually considered to be closely related, but there are infact several key areas of overlap between these fields. Behavior factors determine the choice of foods in the diet, and any attempt to change dietary patterns must necessarily involve the central nervous system and may be associated with mood changes. That diet influences behavior is an ancient human belief. Primitive people attributed friendly and unfriendly feelings to plants and animals and expected these feelings to be transferred to anyone who ate such foods.

In religious teachings, the behavior of mankind was said to change instantly when Eve ate the apple. Solomon, suffering the pangs of love, was confronted with apples. The ancient Greeks proposed that the body is composed of four "humors" - hot, cold, wet, and dry - that control health, feelings, and behavior. Such ideas have carried forth to the present day, when many cultures believe in hot/cold or yin/yang approaches to food and health. Systematic study of cultural influences on food intake began early in this century as anthropologists examined the use of food in isolated cultures and ethnic groups. Even in contemporary times, foods are endowed with magical powers and are believed to symbolize feelings such as those of satisfaction and security.

Behavioral determinants and aspects of eating disorders

Although infants do not begin life with a choice of foods, some of the most obvious reflexes at birth are those associated with eating. Infants learn to associate eating with security and relief from anxiety, tension, and distress. Later, children eat in conformance to cultural and familial standards. These ingrained meanings attached to the roles of food in society suggest reasons that food habits can be changed only with difficulty. Although the choice of certain foods as opposed to others may greatly affect nutritional status, food selection includes multiple environmental, cultural, genetic, social, and sensory variables that interact in complex ways. One exception appears to be an innate preference for foods that are sweet. This preference is acquired in early childhood and continues throughout life. Selection of foods for nutritional or health reasons is a learned behavior.

Infants have not been shown to have an inborn ability to select a balanced, nutritious diet. Variety of foods available has an important effect on food consumption; the more the available foods are varied, the more of them people will eat. Behavior change is a key element in reducing the risk for chronic disease. Eating behaviors are acquired over a lifetime, to change them requires alterations in habits that must be continued permanently - beyond any short-term period of intervention.

Dietary advice is often restrictive and viewed as depriving or unpleasant. It may also be incompatible with cultural or familial standards. Furthermore, environmental factors such as peer pressure, advertising of high-calorie foods and alcoholic beverages may strongly counteract recommended changes. Despite these difficulties, considerable evidence supports the effectiveness of nutrition education in changing dietary intake to reduce risk factors for conditions such as coronary heart disease, diabetes, hypertension, and neurologic disorders.

Bulimia

Bulimia is an eating disorder characterized by recurrent episodes of binge eating in which large amounts of food are consumed over a short period of time. These episodes are usually terminated by abdominal pain, self-induced vomiting, sleep, or the appearance of another person on the scene. Bulimia occurs among persons of normal weight but is present in half the patients with anorexia nervosa. The severity of binge eating ranges from occasional episodes of morbid overeating at a party to the severe form of the disorder, bulimia nervosa, in which the vomiting or purging follows frequent episodes of binge eating.

There are many similarities between persons with anorexia nervosa and bulimia. Both occur primarily in young women, although bulimia occurs in slightly older individuals, both may relate to the current preoccupation with thinness and dieting. The symptoms of depression in the majority of bulimic patients and the presence of biologic markers of depression suggest that bulimia may represent a variant of mood disorder. Treatment of bulimia is cognitive-behavioral and pharmacologic. Behavioral treatment include modification of the behavioral program designed for obese patients and a combination of cognitive-behavioral and insight-oriented approaches.

Pica

Pica is the intentional and compulsive consumption of non-food substances. It occurs worldwide and is common among people of either sex and of all ages and races. Pica is often associated with nutritional deficiencies or toxicities, and is of special concern among young children and pregnant women.

Geophagia is the consumption of earth and clay. Amylophagia is the consumption of starch and paste, and pagophagia is the eating of ice. The fourth category includes the consumption of ash, chalk, antacids, paint chips, plaster, wax, and other substances. People appear to be driven to consume these substances by nutritional deficiencies, but pica is not necessarily correlated with poor nutritional status. The nutritional hazards most frequently associated with pica are lead poisoning and iron deficiency anaemia.

Hypoglycaemia

Hypoglycaemia (low blood sugar) can occur either after a fast (fasting hypoglycaemia) or several hours after the consumption of a meal (reactive hypoglycaemia). Many individuals have symptoms of weakness, confusion, and irritability after eating sugars or other carbohydrate foods. True reactive hypoglycaemia is diagnosed when symptoms of sweating, tremor, anxiety, and irritability occur at the same time as the documented low blood sugar level. Such a diagnosis may indicate the early presence of a disease such as diabetes.

Hyperactive behavior

Hyperactivity is a childhood problem often discussed in relation to nutrition. This condition is characterized by problems of inattention, excessive motion, impulsivity, learning disabilities, and related problems of conduct. Food additives, especially artificial dyes and colours, can cause hyperactivity.

Implications for Public Health Policy

Studies in patients with eating disorders and other chronic disease conditions emphasize the importance of modification of diet-related behavior in these conditions. Although evidence linking dietary caffeine, refined sugars, and food additives to behavioral disorders is uncertain, their elimination from thediet will not impair nutritional status and can be recommended to patients on an individual trial basis.

Maternal and Child Nutrition

Although the precise contribution of nutrition to maternal and infant health cannot yet be distinguished from genetic, environmental, or behavioural factors that affect risk, an inadequate diet during pregnancy increases the probability of a low birth weight (LBW) infant, who, in turn, has an increased risk of mortality. Well-nourished mothers who gain appropriate amounts of weight during pregnancy generally give birth to heavier, healthier babies. The most important factor contributing to the infant mortality rate is a low birth weight - less than 2500 g. Infant deaths and illnesses increase sharply as birth weight declines. LBW infants are at increased risk for developmental handicaps, birth defects, respiratory and other infectious diseases, behaviour problems, and complications of medical interventions. Medical, social, behavioural, and dietary factors before and during pregnancy contribute to the risk for LBW. Dietary factors include an inadequate intake of calories or essential nutrients such as protein, vitamins, and minerals. The more these risk factors are present, the greater the risk to mother and child.

Infants

Immediately after birth, weight is lost, but birth weight is usually regained by the 10th day. After this time, weight increases at a rapid but decelerating rate. Most infants double their birth weight by the age of 4 months and triple it within a year.

Children and Adolescents

The very rapid rate of growth in infancy is followed by slower growth during the preschool and early school-age years. Children become leaner between 6 months and 6 years, after which a gradual increase in fat thickness occurs in both males and females untilpuberty; females have a relatively greater body fat content than males at all stages of development.

Nutritional Needs of Pregnant and Lactating Women

Extra energy and nutrients are needed to support the growth of maternal tissues, and the increased metabolic demands of pregnancy as well as the growth of the fetus and placenta. During lactation, the energy and nutrients provided in the milk, and those required for its production, must be replaced. Maternal pregnancy weight and weight gained during pregnancy are important determinants of infant birth weight. Inadequate weight gain during pregnancy and low prepregnancy weight combined with low weight gain are associated with lower than average infant birth weight and greater risks for fetal or neonatal death and neonatal disease. The RDA for vitamins and minerals for pregnant or lactating women include levels above those for nonpregnant women.

In healthy women with normal pregnancies, vitamin and mineral needs can usually be met by consuming an adequate diet. Supplements, although usually recommended, are not always associated with measurable health improvements in this population. The need for iron is increased during pregnancy, and the National Research Council recommends an iron supplement of 30 to 60 mg per day to prevent depletion of iron stores during pregnancy and lactation. Pregnant women should be evaluated periodically to determine their level of iron stores and should receive supplements when iron stores are low. The RDA for zinc includes a 5 mg per day increment during pregnancy over the 15 mg per day recommended for nonpregnant women. The rate of fetal malformations and other poor outcomes of pregnancy may be higher in populations whee zinc deficiency has been recognized.

Role of Dietary Factors in Child Health

The energy requirements of children are determined by their individual basal metabolic rates, rates of growth, and activity patterns. Therefore, appropriate intakes for children of the same age, sex, and size vary. Children need protein for the maintenance of body tissues, changes in body composition, and synthesis of new muscles. During growth, the protein content of the body increases from about 15 percent at one year to 18 percent by four years, which is also the value for adults. The RDA for protein decreases from 1.8 g per kg per day at one year to 0.8 g per kg per day at 18 years.

Inadequate intakes of vitamins and minerals will be reflected in slow growth rates, inadequate mineralization of bones, and very low reserves of micronutrients. With the relatively low prevalence of clinical signs of vitamin and mineral deficiency in the general population of children, there is no evidence that supplementation is necessary for this group. Although vitamin and mineral supplements increase the quantity of these nutrients in the diet, they have not been shown to improve biochemical indices of nutrient status in children who are already well nourished. For this reason, recommendations for vitamin and mineral supplements target children at high risk, those from socioeconomically deprived families, and those who have poor appetites or eating habits. Preschool children are a nutritionally vulnerable group. Their growth rate is slower than it was in infancy and their nutritional needs in relation to body size proportionately reduced. Thus, they often want and eat relatively little food. Food intake can be reduced even further by the increasing independence (expressed as refusals to eat) and immature feeding skills that are characteristic of very young children.

Parents continue to be the main influence on the food intake of school-aged children, although an increasing proportion of the diet is consumed in schools, day care centres, and fast food restaurants. Between the ages of 4 and 6, children increase the varieties of foods they are willing to eat. Snacks become an important source of calories and nutrients, and may contribute as much as one-third of calories and fat, one-fifth of the protein, and nearly one-half of the carbohydrate 10-year-old children consume. These patterns emphasize the need for parents and schools to provide appropriate meals and snacks and guidance in food choices.

Role of Dietary Factors in Adolescent Health

Energy and nutrient requirements are directly related to the stage and rate of growth, and demands are greatest during the peak velocity of growth. For most nutrients the RDA's are similar to those for adults. The RDA for calcium, 1200 mg per day, is higher for adolescents than for adults and is designed to meet the needs of the adolescent who is growing at the fastest rate. Achieving maximum bone mass during the teens and twenties can reduce the risk of developing osteoporosis later in life. The higher RDA for iron for adolescent males is also related to rapid growth, which is accompanied by increases in blood volume, muscle mass, and iron-containing enzymes. Vitamin requirements are correlated withgrowth demands rather than age.

The growth surge of adolescence demands significant increases in calories and nutrient intake to support the rapid growth rate and increased body size. In early adolescence, children still depend on their parents for food, but by the end of adolescence they are largely independent. Irregular eating patterns are common in adolescence, reflecting this growing independence from the family and the teenager's increasingly busy social life and athletic, academic, and vocational activities. Breakfast or lunch are often skipped or eaten on the run. Snacking is characteristic of this age group and contributes significantly to nutrient intake. These snack foods are often higher in calories, fat and sugar, and lower in vitamins, minerals, and fibre, than foods consumed at family meals. Because lifetime dietary patterns are established during these years, adolescents should be encouraged to choose nutritious foods, to develop good eating habits, and to maintain appropriate levels of physical activity.

3

Balance Diet, its Elements and Sources

Natural Health

Vitamins are essential to growth and health. They help the body to resist disease and body cells to function properly. We have to consider two types of vitamins - water soluble and fat soluble.

The B-complex and vitamin C are water soluble. They cannot be stored in the body in large amounts so must be supplied regularly in the diet. When a dog loses fluids by vomiting or diarrhoea, its vitamins must be replaced.. Overfeeding these water-soluble vitamins does not cause toxicity as excesses are lost in the urine.

Vitamin B1 (thiamine)

— This is very important to dogs.

— Dogs differ genetically in their need for thiamine.

— Metabolic disturbance, exercise and cold housing may increase demand.

— Only small amounts of thiamine are stored in the body.

— Treating meat for hydatids (freezing and boiling) reduces thiamine - it is lost in the thawed water and boiling juices.

The heat of cooking will destroy thiamin. Commercially prepared dog feeds have extra thiamine added to their diets to compensate for cooking losses.

— If you are cooking your own feed recipe, add some yeast tablets to it.

— Feed a dog supplementary thiamine 2-3 times a week.

— Brewer's (not live) yeast and wheat germ are valuable sources.

— Meat and cereals are also good sources.

— A high fat diet contains less thiamine than a high-carbohydrate diet.

Never feed dogs raw fish as some species contain an enzyme (thiaminase) which will make thiamine unavailable. Nervous symptoms may develop leading to paralysis. Cooked fish is safe as thiaminase is destroyed.

Vitamin B-complex

These include riboflavin (Vit B2), niacin pyridoxin (Vit B6), pantothenic acid, biotin, folic acid, and vitamin B12. The best supplies are in wheat germ, brewer's yeast, liver and the organ and muscle meats. Under normal feeding there should be no problems, but egg white and sulpha drugs can make them unavailable. "Black tongue" is a defect of the mucous membranes caused by a niacin deficiency. Poor blood clotting can be caused by folic acid deficiency. Riboflavin shortage can cause slow growth, poor appetite and low fertility.

Vitamin C

Plenty of this is synthesised by the dog to meet its needs.

Fat-soluble vitamins

These vitamins (A, D, E and K) need fat to be transported and absorbed by the body. So if the fat metabolism of the dog is upset, then a vitamin deficiency may occur.

Get veterinary advice when supplementing fat soluble vitamins as excess builds up and is stored in the body fat and can lead to problems.

— Liver, kidney, muscle fat and fish liver oil are good sources.

— Handle fats with care - the vitamins are lost if the fat goes rancid.

— Vitamin A deficiency results in deafness, nervousness, diarrhoea, retarded growth and partial loss of vision (night blindness).

Excess vitamin A will lead to bone deformities.

Vitamin D deficiency results in rickets (bowed legs) and enlarged joints seen in pups growing quickly (knobbly knees and splayed feet) An excess of vitamin D will lead to over calcification of bones and soft tissue such as heart, lungs and muscles.

Vitamin E deficiency causes pups to be born weak or dead. Can lead to muscular dystrophy and hear muscle damage.

Vitamin K deficiency reduces blood-clotting ability. It's rare in normal diets.

Minerals

There is a range of minerals needed for various functions of the body. They are used in the skeleton (bones and teeth), muscles, glands, body fluids and for correct functioning of the cells. Deficiency problems are easily avoided if you feed a balanced diet. Commercial diets these days provide more of these minerals than are needed by the dog so there are no concerns. Important minerals are:

— Calcium

— Phosphorus

— Magnesium
— Sodium
— Chlorine
— Potassium

If you ever see a feed analysis (eg. on the bag of purchased dog feed), you'll see a component called "ash". This is what's left after the feed has been burned to measure the heat or energy released. All the mineral components are in the remaining ash part.

Calcium and phosphorus

These two minerals are closely linked in the health of the dog and are very important. We need to consider not only the amount fed, but also the ration between them. This is referred to as the Ca:P ratio. The general recommended ratio in a good diet for a mature dog is between 1.2 and 1.4 parts of calcium(Ca) to 1.2 part of phosphorus (P). Meat has a Ca:P ratio of about 1:10 while liver has a 1:40 ratio. Liver is also a good source of vitamins A and D which tends to modify the effects of a calcium deficiency Calcium deficiency is most common bone disease in dogs caused by poor feeding. It can happen by a shortage of calcium or an excess of phosphorus in the diet upsetting the Ca:P ratio. You won't fix a deficiency by throwing your dog a few bones to chew! Never feed a dog cooked bones, fish bones or chicken bones.

Watch out for meat rich diets which are high in P and low in Ca. When the body tries to balance up the Ca:P ratio, loss of bone mass which results in pain in the bones, joints and muscles can occur. Lameness and a tendency for bones to fracture is seen , and in pups you get poor tooth development and sore and swollen joints. Pups should be reared on a diet with a Ca:P ratio of 1.4:1. You can ensure this by adding bone flour or calcium phosphate at 15-20g/kg of dry food to the diet of a large rapidly growing pup

Sodium

The dog will get plenty of this in its diet as salt (sodium chloride), and often the concern is feeding too much. Providing plenty of water is essential to avoid toxicity by feeding too much. In very hot conditions, the dog may need extra salt.

Magnesium and potassium

These are important to the dog and can be best provided by feeding liver, heart, or muscles in general.

Trace elements

Some components of the dog's diet are only needed in very small or "trace" amounts - hence the name trace elements. Excess intake of some of these can cause poisoning, or too much of one can affect absorption of another.

The way to avoid any problems is to feed a good balanced diet. Seek veterinary advice if you feel the need to add extra supplements.

Water

Water is not a strictly a nutrient but it's essential to life. Muscle for example contains 80% water, fat 20-30% and bone in a young animal 70-80%. Animals will survive for a long time without feed but will soon dehydrate without water. Blood, which transports all the digested nutrients around the body, is largely water as is the lymph which finally bathes the cells in nutrients. Blood and lymph then carry the waste products away from the body cells and tissues for excretion. Water is the main constituent of all digestive juices and gland secretions. It's also a product of digestion when foodstuffs are broken down in the body to produce heat and energy. Dogs should always have a clean water available at their kennels. There will be a large variation in how much a dog will drink depending on its work load and so on. Don't let a dog drink large amounts of water just before or just after strenuous work. Frequent small drinks during work are best and will increase endurance. But it's hard to stop the dog diving into the creek on a hot day and trying to drink it dry!

The Nutrient Balance Approach to Obesity

There are several models that can be used to develop a framework for understanding obesity. One could use a public health model in which the interaction between food, an environmental agent, and the host are examined. Alternatively one could use a genetic model in which the interaction of genetic factors and environmental agents are used to explain obesity. In addition, behavioral models, metabolic models and set-point models might also be used. A nutrient balance model for the control of nutrient stores, obesity is viewed as a homeostatic failure of nutrient balance resulting from a failure of nutrients to stimulate the sympathetic nervous system. It is hoped that this approach will provide a useful system for understanding the development of obesity.

The Nutrient Balance Model

A regulated or controlled system has several components. First, there is a controller located in the brain. Second, there is a controlled system consisting of intake, digestion, absorption, storage and metabolism of the nutrients in food. Third, there are feedback elements which tell the controller about the state of the controlled system, and finally, there are the efferent control mechanisms which modulate food intake and energy expenditure.

The Controlled System

The normal adult human being contains approximately 140,000 kcal of energy in body fat. This is some six times the quantity of energy that is stored in protein. By comparison, the quantity of carbohydrate is minute, equivalent to only 800 kcal, which includes glycogen stores from liver, kidney, muscle and other tissues plus the glucose that circulates in the blood. Individuals eating 2000 kcal, of which 40% is carbohydrate, will take in an amount of carbohydrate each day comparable to their total body stores. In contrast, average daily protein intake is only a little over 1% of total stores and fat intake is considerably less than 1%. It should not be surprising, therefore, that in studies of nutrient balance in experimental animals, that changes in carbohydrate balance from day to day reciprocally affected carbohydrate intake on the subsequent day. For fat balance, on the other hand, the day to day relationship was very weak.

There are two major pathways for absorption of digested food from the gut. One of these pathways is through the lacteals which transport triglycerides packaged as chylomicrons. These enter the venous circulation and are cleared in the periphery by hydrolysis of triglycerides catalyzed by the enzyme lipoprotein lipase. The other pathway for absorption of glucose and amino acids as well as short chain fatty acids is through the portal vein directly to the liver. The nutrients that enter the controlled system can be stored, converted to heat through metabolism or used for work. In addition, small quantifies can be excreted in the urine as the end-products of metabolism of amino acids. The resting metabolism of human beings is directly related to the amount of fat free or lean body mass. In addition, there is an important familial component in energy expenditure. Physical work accounts for approximately 1/3 of the energy expended. That body weight and energy stores are well regulated over short intervals in most individuals has been suggested in a number of studies. For most adults the sensitivity of the system for changes is less than 1% per year.

An analysis of this regulatory control system suggests the following concepts:

— Each major nutrient may be regulated separately.

— The time required to achieve balance for each nutrient varies as a function of the amount ingested each day in relation to the total body stores of that nutrient. Thus, becoming obese by eating a high-carbohydrate diet would appear to be more difficult than with a high-fat diet because the body storage system for carbohydrate as glycogen is limited. Although excess carbohydrate can be converted to fatty acids, this is an energetically expensive transformation. Body fat stores, on the other hand, are many times larger than daily fat intake, implying a much greater capacity for fat storage and a much longer time constant to achieve balance.

— Achievement of nutrient balance requires that the net oxidation of each nutrient equals the average composition of the macronutrients in the diet. That is, ingestion of a high-fat diet requires greater oxidation of fat than a low-fat diet

— There are major differences between individuals in the capacity to increase rapidly the oxidation of fat after beginning a high-fat diet. Much of this difference is genetic.

— Physical training can increase oxidation of fatty acids by muscle, and thus, regular aerobic exercise might reduce the tendency to become obese when eating a high-fat diet.

— The regulation of nutrient stores is subject to positive and negative feedback signals for each component that operates through the central controller.

Nutrient intake plays a variable role in the development of obesity in man and animals. At one extreme are the types of obesity depicted in stone age carvings. Obesity in these people develops regardless of the type of diet available. In these instances, genetic factors probably play an important role since in experimental animals with a genetic tendency to obesity the type of diet is unimportant in its development. At the other extreme are those types of obesity where dietary composition is central to its appearance. These include a high-fat diet and access to sweetened beverages containing sucrose and diets with an abundance of highly palatable foods. Any of these types of dietary obesity can be controlled by changing diets along with restraint in levels of food intake.

Afferent Feedback Singlas

The brain receives information. for regulating nutrient balance from several sources. Afferent signals can be transmitted over the somatic sensory nervous system, via the autonomic nervous system or through the bloodstream.

Sensory Signals: The sight and smell of food are important signals for identifying potential sources of food and initiating food intake. Along with the texture and taste of food in the mouth, the sensory cues about the quality of food can serve as positive feedback signals for initiating food ingestion as well as negative feedback signals which eventually slow down, terminate or abort an eating incident. The ability of most animals to avoid foods that have previously made them sick, a phenomenon known as bait-shyness, is an example of these afferent sensory signals integrated with a central learning system.

Gastrointestinal Signals: Information from food in the gastrointestinal tract can be initiated by one of three mechanisms:

- first--gastrointestinal distension,
- second--release of gastrointestinal hormones when nutrients act directly on the gastrointestinal tract and
- third--through the effects of absorbed nutrients.

Both gastric and intestinal distension are mechanisms for terminating meals by negative feedback via the nervous system. The vagus nerve is probably the principal afferent sensory relay for this type of information. Several gastrointestinal hormones have been implicated in the inhibition of feeding. The one studied most prominently is cholecystokinin (CCK). It has been demonstrated that intraperitoneal injections of CCK decrease food intake in hungry rats as well as inhibit sham feeding in rats and monkeys. Furthermore, it has been demonstrated that the sequence of events associated with a response to CCK is similar to that of spontaneous postprandial satiety. One suggestion for the effect of CCK is that it acts on antral CCK receptors (CCK-A) receptors by constricting the pylorus and enhancing gastric distension. Peripheral information generated by CCK may be important in producing satiety since vagotomy and lesions in the central vagal connections (nucleus of the tractus solitarius), the ventromedial hypothalamus and the paraventricular nucleus will block the effect of CCK. Bombesin nd the N-terminal pentapeptide from procolipase may also be signals produced in the gastrointestinal tract that inhibit feeding.

Nutrient Signals: Nutrient signals may also act on the liver or brain to initiate satiety. Glucose injected into the portal circulation decreases vagal afferent firing rate, probably through acting on hepatic glucose receptors. Glucose may also act directly on the central nervous system since this nutrient is the major source of fuel for this organ. This glucose may serve to regulate the binding of appetite-suppgressing drugs in the hypothalamus.

Vitamins

Vitamins are organic substances functioning to facilitate an essential biochemical reaction necessary for growth, vitality and the normal functioning of our bodies. We must obtain them from our diet or take them in the form of dietary supplements, that are usually derived from plant and animal products. Crucial to the definition of a vitamin is that lack of it produces a specific deficiency syndrome, and supplying it cures that deficiency. It is almost impossible to sustain a healthy way of life by taking only synthetic supplements and not following a good eating plan. Supplements should be taken only with some nutrition knowledge or the guidance of a nutritionist and dietitian.

Many vitamins and minerals can be toxic if taken in excess. Often there are sufficient vitamins in your diet, thus by taking supplements toxicity may occur. Symptoms include hair loss, blurred vision, bone pain, fatigue and headaches. The best way of obtaining a healthy balance of vitamins is by eating a large variety of different foods. One should try not to limit their diet to a few delicacies. Try out new dishes, be adventurous.

Fat-Soluble Vitamins: The fat-soluble vitamins are vitamins A, D, E, and K. These vitamins are absorbed, transported, metabolized and stored along with fat. The fat soluble vitamins function as regulators for specific metabolic activity.

Water-soluble Vitamins: The water-soluble vitamins include vitamin C, and those of the B-complex group: biotin, folate, niacin, pantothenic acid, riboflavin, thiamin, vitamin B6, and vitamin B12. They function mainly as coenzymes.

Vitamin Supplements

No data have yet been published to demonstrate that healthy people eating a well balanced diet need any vitamin supplements. A well balanced diet means that what one has eaten during the day should include a wide variety of foods from each of the five food groups (fruit, vegetables, bread and grains, meat and milk). Except in pregnancy, where supplementation of certain vitamins may be recommended, there are no reports of normal persons eating a well balanced diet developing vitamin deficiency diseases. The proper role of vitamin supplementation is in the treatment of deficienc in patients who have inadequate intake, disturbed absorption, or increased requirements because of an increased destruction or excretion. Mega-dose therapy is the treatment with daily quantities of a vitamin or vitamins substantially above the Recommended Dietary Allowances (RDA) of the Food and Nutrition Board. The RDAs are the levels of intake of essential nutrients considered to be adequate to meet the known nutritional needs of all healthy persons.

Vitamins, like many other substances, may be toxic when taken in large quantities. Large doses of nicotinic acid frequently cause flushing and itching, liver damage, dermatoses, elevations of serum glucose concentration and peptic ulceration may occur. Prolonged excessive intake of vitamin D can cause anorexia, nausea, weakness, weight loss, hypertension, anemia, hypercalcemia, irreversible renal failure, and death. Vitamin E in large doses antagonises the action of vitamin A and also causes headaches, nausea, fatigue, blurred vision, inflammation of the mouth, chapping of the lips, gastrointestinal disturbances, muscle weakness, low blood sugar, increased bleeding tendency, and degenerative changes. The comments that vitamin doses in excess of the RDA may produce "optimal" health are pure speculation, unsupported by any facts in human metabolism, and contradicted by the toxicity of vitamin and mineral doses in excess of the RDA. "More is better" is a slogan, not science. More is sometimes better, sometimes worse, but always costlier.

Vitamin A (Retinol, Carotene)

Vitamin A is fat soluble, it is an antioxidant and occurs in two forms - retinol and carotene. The RDA [Food and Nutrition Board, National Academy of Sciences - National Research Council - Recommended Dietaty Allowances.] for adults is 1000 micrograms RE (Retinol Equivalents. 1 RE = 1 microgram retinol or 6 micrograms β-carotene).

The allowances, expressed as average daily intakes over time, are intended to provide for individual variations among most normal persons as they live in the United States under usual environment stresses. The RDA's given are the higher of adult males or females, for more precise data refer to table at the end of Part 1. Because vitamin A and carotene exist in more than one chemical form, and because they are not equally active, it is usual to give the name retinol to the pure vitamin A. Thus the total vitamin A activity of a food, its retinol equivalent, is determined by how much it contains of retinol, chemicals very similar to retinol but not as active, and a range of carotenes also of varying activity. Vitamin A maintains the skin and mucous membranes. Promotes growth, strong bones, healthy skin, hair, teeth and gums. Builds up resistance to respiratory infections and shortens the duration of diseases.

It counteracts night blindness and aids in the treatment of many eye disorders.

Night blindness is an early symptom of a deficiency of vitamin A. In a dozen case-control and cohort studies, intakes of fruits and vegetables containing carotenoids has been associated with a reduced risk of lung cancer. In contrast little relationship has been found between intake of preformed vitamin A (retinol) and this disease. Available data thus strongly support the hypothesis that dietary carotenoids reduce the risk of lung cancer, but the data also are compatible with the possibility that some other factor in these foods is responsible for the lower risk. The recommendation to eat a variety of fruits and vegetables is reasonable, but leaves much to chance; if ß-carotene is the anticancer agent, intake of specific fruits and vegetables should be advised. The best natural sources are green leafy vegetable tops, carrots, red peppers, sweet potatoes, yellow fruits, apricots, fish-liver oil and eggs.

Vitamin A is one of the few vitamins in which excess produces definite and severe effects. Toxic symptoms can occur with intake exceeding 100 000 IU's daily. Hypervitaminosis A leads to loss of appetite, a dry, itchy skin often with peeling, intense headaches and an enlarged liver. Recovery is fairly rapid when intake is reduced.

Vitamin B1 (Thiamine)

Vitamin B1 is water soluble like all the B vitamins. It is easily lost and must be replaced daily. The RDA for adults is 1.5 milligrams. Thiamine prevents and cures beriberi, a disease of the nervous system. It aids growth, maintains normal carbohydrate metabolism and nervous system functioning. It helps alleviate stress conditions, anxiety and trauma.

The best natural sources are dried yeast, spirulina, whole wheat, oats, peanuts, soybeans, green vegetables and milk. This vitamin is not toxic, it is easily excreted from the body and not stored. It is destroyed by heat, caffeine, alcohol and cigarette smoke.

Vitamin B2 (Riboflavin)

Vitamin B2 is not stored and must be replaced daily. The RDA for adults is 1.7 milligrams. Essential for normal cell growth, helps to metabolize carbohydrates, fats and proteins. Benefits vision and eye fatigue, promotes healthy skin, nails and hair. Eliminates sores in mouth, on lips and tongue. The best natural sources are milk, yeast, cheese, sea vegetables, leafy green vegetables, mushrooms, fish and eggs. There are no known toxic effects. It is destroyed by light, alcohol and sulfur drugs.

Vitamin B3 (Niacin, Nicotinic Acid)

Niacin is a component of an enzyme and can be produced by the body, some of the amino acid tryptophane is converted into niacin. The RDA for adults is 19 milligrams. It is necessary for a wide variety of body processes, reduces high blood pressure, lowers cholesterol levels and prevents pellagra. Without niacin, thiamine and riboflavin cannot function properly. The best natural sources are lean meat, whole wheat, tuna, anchovy, yeast, eggs, peanuts and avocados. Niacin is not toxic but people with peptic ulcers or diabetes should consult a doctor before taking supplements greater than 100 milligrams.

Vitamin B5 (Pantothenic Acid)

It is known in other forms - Calcium Pantothenate and Panthenol. The RDA for adults is 7 milligrams. It is necessary for the utilization of other nutrients and maintaining normal growth and development of the nervous system, as well as for the metabolism of fat and sugars. The best natural sources are fish, whole grains, wheat germ, green vegetables and brewers yeast. There are few known toxic effects, but very large doses have been known to produce lack of co-ordination in movement and impairment of sensation. It is destroyed by heat, caffeine and alcohol.

Vitamin B6 (Pyridoxine)

B6 has three metabolic forms pyridoxine, pyridoxal and pyridoxamine. The RDA for adults is 2.0 milligrams. It is essential in amino acid metabolism, is required for the absorption of B12 and for the production of antibodies and red blood cells. The best natural sources are bananas, brewer's yeast, wheat germ, green and red peppers, nuts, molasses and eggs. Intake should be increased with diets high in protein. Daily doses of over 500 mg should be avoided. Doses over 2 g can lead to neurological disorders. Food processing techniques, canning and alcohol can deplete vitamin B6.

Vitamin B12 (Cyancobalimin, Cobalamin)

B12 contains mineral elements - cobalt. The RDA for adults is 2.0 micrograms. Cobalamins are necessary for protein and fatty acid metabolism and the production of red blood cells. It maintains a healthy nervous system and improves concentration and memory. The best natural sources are clams, oysters, beef, eggs and dairy products. It is not found in many plant products except certain soya products, tempeh and sea vegetables. If you are a strict vegetarian you will need to take B12 supplements. Although, people who have diets high in protein need more B12. A deficiency can cause pernicious anemia. B12 is not easily absorbed and needs to be combined with calcium for proper absorption. It is destroyed by sunlight, alcohol and sleeping pills. There have been no reports of B12 toxicity.

Vitamin B15 (Pangamic Acid, Pangamate, Calcium Pangamate)

Pangamic acid has not had much research done on it in the USA, but has been approved in Russia and used by athletes to enhance performance. Pangamic acid is a label not a product. The pills contain anything the seller chooses to put in them. The Food and Drug Administration contend that "B15" is essentially an untested food additive which is not generally recognized by the scientific experts as safe for human consumption. Pangamate was prohibited within Canada for almost two decades. Because of these facts, any physician who prescribes it should first get informed consent from his or her patients after informing them that it is not a vitamin, has no known nutrient value, no known value in the long-term treatment of any disease, that its safety has not been established, and that it may be mutagenic (cancer causing).

The allegations that pangamic acid is an antioxidant, protects against pollutants, increases the life span of cells, relieves symptoms of asthma and lowers blood cholesterol levels, as well as that it stops the craving for alcohol and protects the liver from cirrhosis are anecdotal and testimonial stories rather than studies. The authors often claim spectacular results from "pangamic acid" without identifying which of the many chemicals and chemical combinations which go by that name they are using. Without distinguishing drug effect from the placebo, and without reporting any evaluation of patients for short-term or long-term toxic effects.

Vitamin B17 (Laetrile)

Laetrile is the trademark of a compound of two parts glucose and one part cyanide. There is no vitamin B17, "B17" is a tradename created for laetrile by a laetrile proponent. It is naturally present in the kernels of apricot pits and a number of other stone fruits and nuts. There is no RDA but doses vary from 0.25 g to 1.0 g a day. It is believed to have cancer controlling and preventative properties. Apparently normal cells can tolerate small quantities of cyanide but cancer cells succumb to it. Cyanide has no value in sustaining human life. In small amounts it injures, in larger amounts it kills. No law prevents promoters from trade-naming nutritionally worthless or poisonous substances.

Cyanide is rapidly absorbed from the intestine and diffuses throughout the body, knocking out respiration in cells. Eating about 25 apricot kernels can cause headaches, dizziness, nausea, drowsiness, a sharp fall in blood pressure, breathing difficulties, coma and death. There have been documented cases of people dying after taking as few as five laetrile tablets. Not more than 1.0 gram should be taken at any one time.

Vitamin C (Ascorbic Acid)

Ascorbic acid is water soluble and is easily lost from the body. The RDA for adults is 60 milligrams. It is important for the growth and repair of body tissue cells, bones, gums and teeth. It fights bacterial infections, protects Vitamin A, some of the B vitamins and vitamin E from oxidation and is necessary for the use of iron and oxygen in the body. People who lack this vitamin may have sore gums and bleeding under the skin. It helps to reduce blood cholesterol levels, aids in preventing bacterial and viral infections, and prevents and cures scurvy. The best natural sources are citrus fruits, hot chili peppers, broccoli, tomatoes, green leafy vegetables, and sweet potatoes. Vitamin C is non toxic but people with peptic ulcers, might hemorrhage and should consult a doctor before taking supplements. It is lost through water, destroyed by cooking, heat, light and smoking.

Vitamin D (Calciferol)

It is a fat soluble vitamin and can be produced in the skin with exposure to sunlight. The RDA for adults is 10 micrograms or 400 IU. (as cholecalciferol. 10 micrograms cholecalciferol = 400 IU of vitamin D.] It regulates calcium and phosphate metabolism. Aids the assimilation of vitamin A and helps the treatment of conjuctivites and rickets. The best natural sources are sardines, herring and dairy products. It is produced by interaction with sunlight and oils (cholesterol) in the skin. It can be toxic with doses of over 5000 IU daily. In smog conditions or when activities reduce exposure to sunlight vitamin D intake should be increased.

Vitamin E (Tocopherol)

Vitamin E is the term used for eight naturally occurring, fat-soluble nutrients called tocopherols - alpha, beta, gamma, delta, epsilon, zeta, eta and theta. Alpha-Tocopherol is essential, has the highest biological activity, and predominates in many species. The RDA for adults is 10 IU. (Designated according to its biological activity in International Units (IU). With this vitamin 1 IU = 1 mg Alpha Tocopherol Equivalents). In human beings, vitamin E is the most important fat-soluble antioxidant. It prevents the potentially harmful oxidation of fat compounds and enhances the functioning of vitamin A. It is an antipollutant for the lungs. It helps the healing of scar tissue when taken internally and also when applied externally.

The best natural sources are wheat germ, whole grains, vegetable oils, soya beans, nuts, apples, apricots and green vegetables. Vitamin E deficiency may cause anemia, as a result of red blood cell destruction and neurological dysfunction, myopathies, and diminished erythrocyte life span. New clinical evidence from heavy drinkers suggests that alcohol may increase oxidation of Alpha-Tocopherol. Increased demand has also been observed in premature infants and patients with malabsorption. It is generally non toxic but some evidence suggests that large intakes may cause increased levels of blood cholesterol and lipids. It can oxidize within a few months of being manufactured, so supplements should not be stored for more than a few months. It is destroyed by heat, freezing, food processing, chlorine and iron.

Vitamin K (Menadione)

Vitamin K is a fat soluble vitamin usually formed in the body by intestinal bacteria but also available from some plant and animal sources. The RDA for adult males is 80 micrograms. Its primary function is to control the rate of blood clotting and prevent internal bleeding. The best natural sources are all leafy green vegetables, cauliflower, brussel sprouts, broccoli, soybean oil, kelp, cereal grain products, fruits and yoghurt.

Vitamin K deficiency has been reported in patients treated with antibiotics and placed on poor diets after surgery. A deficiency can cause bleeding disorders. Doctors sometimes give women vitamin K before childbirth to prevent bleeding in the newborn baby. Babies do not have enough intestinal bacteria to produce adequate amounts of the vitamin until they are about 2 weeks old. No toxicity symptoms have been recorded from natural forms but supplementation of synthetic vitamin K exceeding 500 mcg is not recommended as it can cause anemia and kernicterus, a condition characterized by jaundice.

Biotin

Biotin is a member of the B complex family and is water soluble. The RDA for adults is 100 micrograms. It is essential for the metabolism of fats and the synthesis of ascorbic acid. It maintains a healthy skin and helps prevent baldness and hair from turning grey. The best natural sources are soya beans, brown rice, nuts, fruit, brewer's yeast and milk. It can be synthesized by intestinal bacteria. It is not toxic. Avidin, a substance found in egg white prevents biotin absorption. Sulfur drugs, food processing and alcohol destroy biotin.

Choline

Choline is a cofactor of the B vitamins. There is no RDA but the average adult diet contains between 500 milligrams to 900 milligrams a day. Choline exists in combination with phospholipids which make up part of the brain and spinal cord tissue. These compounds are called lecithins. It is essential for growth and is involved in fat transport and in carbohydrate and protein metabolism. It participates in the metabolism of fat and emulsifies cholesterol, helping to control the build up in arteries. It aids in the treatment of Alzheimer's disease and helps to remove drugs and poisons from your system. It is also the precursor of acetylcholine, which is involved in the transmission of nerveimpulses. It is crucial for normal brain functioning and memory. It goes directly into the brain cells and produces a chemical that aids memory. The best natural sources are soya lecithin, green leafy vegetables, yeast and wheat germ. There is no known toxicity. It is destroyed by sulfur drugs, food processing and alcohol.

Folic Acid (Folate, Folacin)

Folic acid is a cofactor of the B complex vitamins. The RDA for adults is 200 micrograms. Folate is essential for cell growth because of its involvement in nucleic acid and protein synthesis, and for the formation of red blood cells and protein metabolism. It protects the body against intestinal parasites and food poisoning. Maintains a healthy skin and helps in the treatment of anemia. Megaloblastic anemia caused by folate deficiency is a major problem in world health, especially among pregnant women and patients with malabsorption or alcoholism.

The best natural sources are raw leafy vegetables, fruit, carrots, torula yeast, avocados, beans and whole wheat. Consumption of fresh fruit and green leafy vegetables daily will ensure against dietary folate deficiency. In doses of up to 5 mg a day there has been no sign of toxicity. It is easily lost in boiling water, sunlight, food processing, heat and by taking sulfur drugs. A heavy drinker also needs to increase folic acid intake.

Inositol

Inositol is a cofactor of the B complex vitamins. There is no RDA but the average adult gets about 1 gram per day in their diet. It works with choline in the metabolism of fat and cholesterol. It is essential for the proper conduction of nerve impulses, lowers cholesterol levels, promotes healthy hair and prevents balding. The best natural sources are lecithin, brewer's yeast, lima beans, peanuts, raisins, wheat germ, cabbage, cantaloupe, grapefruit and molasses. It is not toxic but is destroyed by sulfur drugs, food processing, alcohol and coffee.

PABA (Para-aminobenzoic Acid)

PABA is another member of the B complex family of vitamins. There is no RDA but about 100 milligrams is usually included in B complex supplements. It helps in the assimilation of protein and pantothenic acid. It is important for normal skin and hair growth. It can protect you against sunburn, prevent wrinkles, reduce the pain of burns and restore grey hair to its natural color. The best natural sources are whole grains, wheat germ, brewer's yeast, rice and molasses. Non toxic, but high doses over a long period of time may cause nausea and vomiting.

Minerals

Much attention is given to the necessities of vitamins for good health, but the role of minerals is as important. Even if one mineral is lacking the body can not function properly. Minerals are divided into two groups - macro elements and trace elements. They combine with vitamins, form enzymes and are necessary for almost every physiological process. Minerals are found in a broad range of plant and animal foods, as well as in drinking water.

It is not always apparent what the function of minerals are and year by year new minerals are being included in the list of essentials. Like vitamins the best way to overcome this problem is by including a very wide range of foods in your diet.

Calcium

Calcium is the most abundant mineral in the body. The RDA for adults is 1200 milligrams. About 99% is found in the bones and teeth. Calcium also has a role to play in the regulation of various body functions including the cardiovascular and nervous systems. It keeps your heart beating regularly, alleviates insomnia and helps to metabolize iron. The best natural sources are sea vegetables Wakame: 1300, Arame: 1170, Kelp: 1093, (Mg per 100g). Taken from Vegetables from the Sea by Teruko & Seibin Arasaki] , low-fat yogurt, skim milk, beans, tofu, sesame seeds, nuts, sardines with bones, salmon and green vegetables.

Calcium absorption is hindered by the presence of oxalate s in the food. Calcium absorbability of kale (a low-oxalate vegetable) was compared with that of milk in 11 normal women. Absorption of calcium was excellent in all subjects. In 9 of the 11 women, kale calcium absorbability was higher than that of milk calcium. For optimal calcium absorption, a proper amount of vitamin D is needed each day. This can be obtained from fortified milk and cereals, or 15 minutes to an hour of midday sunshine. It appears there is a threshold of calcium intake, below which skeletal reserves may be used to meet daily calcium needs. Studies show that loss of estro prompts rapid loss of bone mineral, especially from the spine, regardless of calcium intake. Intakes over 2000 milligrams per day may lead to hypercalcemia, induce constipation, and inhibit the intestinal absorption of iron, zinc, and other essential minerals.

Chromium

It is difficult to estimate the chromium requirement, but a range of 50 micrograms to 200 micrograms per day is tentatively recommended. Trivalent chromium is required for maintaining normal glucose metabolism. Evidence shows that chromium improves glucose tolerance. Diabetes and coronary heart disease are associated with low chromium concentrations in human tissue. The chemical forms of chromium in foods are not known with certainty, but the bioavailability of chromium compounds has been found to be high in brewer's yeast, shell fish, whole wheat bread and mushrooms. An increased incidence of bronchial cancer has been associated with exposure to dusts containing chromate. But the carcinogenicity of certain chromates bears no relevance to the nutritional role of non toxic trivalent chromium.

Copper

Because of the uncertainty of quantitive human requirements, it is not possible to establish an RDA. 1.5 milligrams to 3.0 milligrams per day has been recommended as a safe and adequate range of dietary copper intake for adults. Copper is an essential nutrient, necessary for extensive body functions. It converts iron to hemoglobin , is essential for the utilization of vitamin C and stops the degeneration of the nervous system. In a study of 10 men who got less than half the suggested copper intake for 6 weeks, four of them responded with a significant increase in cholesterol.

The best natural sources are shell fish, sea vegetables, nuts, seeds, beans and peas. It is found abundantly in tap water because of contamination from copper pipes. Toxicity from dietary sources is extremely rare, but supplementation should be avoided as an excess can lower zinc levels, produce insomnia, hair loss and depression.

Iodine

Approximately 1 mcg per kilogram of body weight is required. The RDA for adults is 150 micrograms. Iodine is an essential component of the thyroid hormones thyroxine and triiodothyronine. It is almost entirely used by the thyroid gland. The thyroid gland controls metabolism, proper growth, helps burn up excess fat and gives you more energy. Deficiency of dietary iodine may result in decreased synthesis of the iodine-containing thyroid hormones. This can lead to cretinism and mental retardation. Iodine intake consistently lower than 50 mcg per day usually leads to thyroid hypertrophy (ie. endemic goiter). In addition, epidemiological and experimental studies suggest that endemic goiter predisposes to cancer of the thyroid.

The best natural sources are seafoods and sea vegetables (kelp, arame and kombu). Iodized salt is a regular source, providing about 75 mcg per gram. Individuals who are sensitive to iodine may react to excessive exposure with iododerma, fever, salivary gland enlargement, visual problems and/or other symptoms. Death from severe forms of iododerma has been reported. Acute responses to the ingestion or injection of large doses of an iodine-containing solution include cardiovascular collapse, convulsions, and asthma attacks.

Adverse effects of iodine have also been reported from dietary supplements, including seaweed extracts, vitamin and mineral preparations. Goiter caused by high iodine intakes has been registered in Japan. The response to excess iodine is variable. Some individuals tolerate large intakes without side effects, whereas others may respond adversely to levels close to recommended intakes. Those who are most likely to respond adversely are those living in endemic goiter areas or for other reasons have habitually had a low intake of iodine, and those who are sensitive to iodine.

The maximum tolerable level of iodine appears to range from 200 mcg per day to 1000 mcg per day. These levels of intake are possible from diets that include milk, iodized salt, seaweed and products containing the red food coloring erythrosine which has high levels of iodine. Generally, iodine intakes by the majority of the population in the USA is considered safe and adequate.

Iron

Iron is a constituent of hemoglobin. Body iron content is regulated by the amount absorbed. The absorption is influenced by body stores and by the amount and type of iron in ingested foods. The RDA for adults is 15 milligrams. It is a vital component of many enzymes, it can promote resistance to disease and prevent fatigue. A trend toward reduced risk of melanoma was observed by Stryker et al when iron intake was increased. A deficiency can cause anemia, resulting in impaired concentration, reduced physical performance and work capacity, and decrease immune function. Ascorbic acid is necessary for the proper assimilation of iron. The best natural sources of iron are sea vegetables, clams, cockles, mussels, oysters, yeast, molasses, beans, nuts, seeds and cereals. Tea, coffee, bran and phytates decrease iron absorption. There are no reported cases of toxicity from foods but iron poisoning may occur from ingesting large amounts of medicinal iron supplements.

Magnesium

Magnesium is known as the antistress mineral. The RDA for adults is 350 milligrams. Many biochemical and physiological processes require magnesium. It is necessary for vitamin C and calcium metabolism. It keeps teeth healthy, brings relief from indigestion and can aid in fighting depression. More than 300 enzymes are known to be activated by magnesium. It controls cellular metabolism and maintains electrical potentials of nerve and muscle membranes for the transmission of impulses across junctions. The best natural sources are whole seeds, nuts, legumes, unmilled grains, green vegetables and bananas. Phytate or fiber may reduce magnesium absorption. Alcohol acts as a diuretic, causing vast quantities to be lost in the urine.

There is no evidence that large dietary intakes of magnesium are harmful to people with normal renal function. In cases of impaired renal function and use of magnesium-containing drugs hypermagnesemia may occur. Symptoms include nausea, vomiting and hypotension. As conditions worsen respiratory depression, coma and asystolic arrest may occur.

Manganese

Because of the lack of manganese deficiency in adults, the current dietary intakes satisfy the needs for this mineral. A provisional daily dietary intake of 5.0 milligrams is recommended. It is necessary for the use of biotin, B1 and C, by the body. It can help eliminate fatigue, improve memory, reduce nervous irritability and assure the proper digestion and utilization of food. A deficiency can cause poor reproductive performance, growth retardation, abnormal formation of bone and cartilage, and an impaired glucose tolerance. The best natural sources are whole grains, cereal products, nuts and green leafy vegetables. Dairy products, meat, fish, and poultry are poor sources.

Toxicity has only been observed with workers exposed to high concentrations of manganese dust or fumes in the air.

Nickel

Nickel is now quite firmly established as an essential nutrient, but no Recommended Dietary Allowance (RDA) or Estimated Safe and Adequate Intake (ESADI) has yet been set for nickel. Research showed that nickel was to be found in blood and tissues at quite consistent levels, that it is associated with DNA and RNA in amounts that suggest physiological significance, and that it occurs also in blood in amounts which appear biologically meaningful.

Nickel is required for normal growth and reproduction in animals, and presumably in human beings as well. It appears to have a role in the modulation of the immune system and in development of the brain. Since brain is depleted in deficiency more than other tissues, the brain and immune system should receive attention in future studies of nickel deficiency. The best sources of nickel include oatmeal, legumes, nuts, cocoa, whole wheat bread, and some leafy vegetables such as kale and lettuce. The danger of nickel toxicity from food appears to be very low, since large amounts of nickel are required to produce any toxic effects through ingestion. But in susceptible people, contact with nickel or nickel salts cause skin irritations.

Chronic exposure at lower levels can cause cancer. Workers exposed to nickel compounds have a higher than normal incidence of cancer of the respiratory tract, particularly of the nasal cavities and lungs. Nickel released from burning tobacco isthought to be responsible for at least part of the carcinogenicity of tobacco smoke. There is no indication of cancer arising from ingestion of the nickel in food.

Phosphorus

The precise requirement for phosphorus is unknown, but a 1 to 1 ratio of calcium to phosphorus will provide sufficient phosphorus for most age groups. The RDA for adults is 1200 milligrams. Phosphorus is an essential component of bone mineral and is necessary for normal bone and tooth structure.

It is involved in almost all physiological chemical reactions. It aids in growth and can lessen the pain of arthritis. The best natural sources are cereal grains, nuts, seeds, meat, poultry and fish. Aluminum hydroxide binds phosphorus, making it unavailable for absorption. An excess of iron and magnesium have the same effect. Phosphorus deficiency results in bone loss and is characterized by weakness, anorexia and pain.

Potassium

Potassium is the principal intercellular cation. There is no RDA but a minimum requirement of 1600 milligrams per day would be adequate. Potassium is of great physiological importance, contributing to the transmission of nerve impulses, the control of skeletal muscle contractility, and the maintenance of normal blood pressure. Deficiency symptoms include weakness, anorexia, nausea, drowsiness and irrational behavior. Potassium is found in most foods since it is an essential constituent of all living cells. The richest dietary sources are unprocessed beans, nuts, leafy green vegetables and fruit.

Low blood sugar levels (hypoglycemia), alcohol or smoking cause potassium loss. Acute intoxication (hyperkalemia) càn cause cardiac arrest and prove fatal.

Selenium

The RDA for male adults is 70 micrograms. Selenium plays a role in pancreatic function, in hepatic heme metabolism, and in the immune response. It has a close metabolic interrelationship with the antioxidant vitamin E. Deficiency only occurs simultaneously with a deficiency of vitamin E and can be cured by supplementation of either. It can neutralize certain carcinogens so possibly provide protection from some cancers. The best natural sources of selenium are seafoods, eggs and depending on the selenium content of the soils in which they are grown, grains and seeds.

Sodium

Sodium is the principal cation of extracellular fluid. As the rate of sodium loss can vary under different conditions there is no official RDA, but the minimum daily requirement for healthy adults is 500 milligrams. Sodium is crucial for regulating the membrane potential of cells and is involved in active transport across cell membranes, it is pumped out in exchange for potassium. It helps the nerves and muscles function properly. Sodium is found in abundance in most processed foods thus there is very little chance of a deficiency occurring with the average Western Diet. The best natural sources are salt, shellfish, anchovy, lox, spirulina, wakame, cheese and red or green peppers. The body may be depleted of sodium under extreme conditions of sweating or chronic diarrhea. Excessive intake of sodium can result in edema and hypertension.

Zinc

The RDA is 15 milligrams per day for men and 12 milligrams per day for women. Recent research suggests that men have a higher need for zinc than do women. Thus, it is appropriate that the RDA is sex-specific for zinc. Zinc is an essential trace element that must be supplied in the diet of human beings so that growth and health can be maintained. It is necessary for protein synthesis and the metabolism of vitamin A, it helps the healing process of internal and external wounds, decreases cholesterol deposits and promotes mental awareness. A deficiency can cause loss of appetite, growth retardation and immunological abnormalities. The best natural sources are oysters, nuts, wheatgerm, whole grain products, brewers yeast, meat, eggs, legumes and seeds.

Zinc is more easily absorbed in small amounts than large amounts. Human studies have shown that milk apparently inhibits zinc absorption. Because cow's milk and milk products are the major sources of calcium and higher levels of calcium have been recommended in women to protect against bone loss, this could be a matter for concern. Its bioavailability is reduced by protein or fiber. Smoking and alcohol also decreases the absorption of zinc. Ingestion of zinc supplements exceeding 15 mg per day is not recommended. Toxicity can cause gastrointestinal irritation and vomiting.

Miscellaneous Substances Addictive Drugs

Use of addictive drugs, such as cocaine, marijuana and nicotine, affects food and liquid intake, behavior, taste preference, and body weight. Changes in specific nutrient status and metabolism can also develop; heroin addiction can cause hyperkalemia and morphine use can result in calcium inhibition. Nutrition-related physiological aspects, such as impaired gastrin release, hypercholesterolemia, and hypothermia are also seen with morphine use.

Nutrition-related conditions can affect sensitivity and dependence on drugs and their effects. Diabetes decreases sensitivity and dependence on morphine, protein deprivation produces preferential fat utilization with low cocaine use, and vitamin D deficiency decelerates morphine dependency. During use and/or withdrawal from nicotine, heroin, marijuana, and cocaine, major changes in food selection occur, which results in weight gain or loss. Changes in food selection and consumption caused by cocaine, nicotine, heroin, and marijuana, particularly during drug withdrawal, should be treated by diet modification. The use of specific nutrients (eg., calcium and vitamin D) to modify the withdrawal process or to stimulate health recovery in the addict is unstudied to date, but is a logical direction for the future.

To the extent that alcohol, cocaine or the other drugs of abuse modify nutritional status or food intake, dietary changes cannot be expected to compensate for those changes. Adopting a balanced eating pattern may help renourish an individual and prevent the negative effects of inadequate intake. Tests of specialized supplements with high levels of several vitamins and minerals have shown benefits in increasing compliance and in reducing hunger for drugs during drug cessation treatment. Nutritional changes have been used during the withdrawal or detoxification stage of drug cessation treatment and for renutrition to enhance withdrawal from alcohol and cocaine. Dietary supplementation (particularly of tyrosine and tryptophan) helped restore brain chemicals modified by cocaine or alcohol.

Marijuana

Marijuana has been found to increase food intake in human beings. A single dose of marijuana produced increased appetite in clinical human studies. Increased weight and total caloric intake have been reported in persons who smoked marijuana for 3 to 7 weeks. Foltin et al. found that men who were given two or three marijuana cigarettes during periods between meals significantly increased their daily caloric intake, the total number of eating occasions, and between-meal snacks. A number of symptoms of nutritional deficiency occurred significantly more often in alcohol and marijuana abusers than in nonusers. These included muscle weakness, bleeding gums, fatigue, dyspnea on exertion, indigestion, appetite loss, sore tongue, and low plasma zinc. All subjects had diets that were adequate in nutrients, but abusers ate less fruit, vegetables, and milk and more snack foods than nonusers. Thus, although marijuana use increases appetite and food intake in human beings, the decrease in dietary quality seen in users is accompanied by several signs of nutritional deficiency.

Heroin

In a few reported cases, heroin overdose in human beings was accompanied by severe rhabdomyolysis, destruction of skeletal muscle accompanied by myoglobinemia, which can lead to acute kidney failure. The condition resulted in severe hyperkalemia, probably caused by a rapid efflux of potassium from damaged muscle cells. The associated acute renal failure may exacerbate the hyperkalemia.

Heroin addicts have shown flat glucose tolerance curves, with an exaggerated and delayed insulin response following oral glucose loading. Heroin addicts have a markedly reduced acute insulin response to glucose administered intravenously and have low potassium values. It is clear that heroin alters glucose tolerance and subsequent metabolism, and the severe adverse effects of the drug on skeletal muscle, kidney function, and glucose metabolism are of concern for human users.

The effects of morphine on lipid profiles could have important implications. Its ability to raise levels of insulin and to induce hypoglycemia and hyperglycemia could have important consequences, especially for persons with diabetes. Because coronary heart disease is a leading cause of incapacitating illness and death, the hypercholesterolemic effect of morphine, threefold increase in the atherogenic index and high aortic cholesterol deposition, is of critical interest. Its antagonistic interaction with calcium and vitamin D is also of interest.

Cocaine

Cocaine abuse can lead to food deprivation or nutrient imbalance in human beings. Castro et al. found that young adult cocaine users ate significantly fewer complete/balanced meals per day, and drank more alcohol and coffee, than non users. Within the cocaine group moderate users perceived themselves as less healthy than did light users. Data regarding specific nutritional effects of cocaine use is sparse. However, the well documented medical effects of cocaine, such as increased heart rate, body temperature and metabolic rate, along with feelings of euphoria and increased energy would increase caloric requirements beyond normal. Cocaine also causes decreased appetite and anorexia by inactivation of the feeding center located on the lateral hypothalamus.

The anorexigenic effects of cocaine as well as its metabolism cause deficiencies of most water soluble vitamins. Studies have demonstrated vitamin B6, thiamin and C deficiencies to be common among cocaine users. If the results of food deprivation in monkeys can be extrapolated to human beings, a vicious circle of food deprivation and cocaine abuse can theoretically occur. It is also interesting to note that there was an elevated prevalence rate for anorexia nervosa and bulimia among 259 cocaine abusers compared with nonaddicts.

Nicotine

The role of nicotine, the ingredient of tobacco that causes

dependence, has emerged as a focal point of smoking research. In 1988, nicotine was designated an addictive drug by the US Surgeon General. Within the past decade, a series of objective studies has increased understanding of the relationships between smoking and nicotine with respect to body weight and food intake. Nicotine changes food selection, based on taste, and appears to alter body weight. In addition, nicotine affects the intrauterine growth of fetuses and decreases birth weight of infants born to smoking mothers. Smokers have higher fat intakes, but not higher total energy intakes, than nonsmokers, according to one study. Grunberg and Morse found a significant inverse relationship between cigarette smoking and sugar consumption in an epidemiological study of the US population, which covered a 14 year period. Smokers who were given a choice of bland, salty and sweet foods expressed the least preference for sweets and ate significantly fewer sweets than did non smokers. Body weight in human beings tends to increase after they quit smoking. This is probably due to the increased consumption of sweet foods (particularly chocolate) after quitting.

Alcohol (Ethanol)

Alcohol is of importance to nutrition because it provides energy (7 kcal per gram) and because it can affect the requirements for and the intake, digestion, absorption, transport, storage, metabolism, and excretion of many other nutrients. Once absorbed, alcohol diffuses rapidly across capillary and other cell membranes and is distributed uniformly throughout all extracellular and intracellular body water. It is first metabolized by the liver to acetaldehyde, then to acetate, and finally to carbon dioxide and water. More than 95 percent is oxidized and the remainder is excreted in the urine, feces, perspiration and expired air. Three types of malnutrition may be observed in alcoholics, primary malnutrition due to a decreased intake of nutrients, secondary malnutrition caused by an impairment in the digestion and absorption of nutrients, and tertiary malnutrition due to an alteration in the ability to convert nutrients to their active coenzyme forms, resulting in nutritional complications that potentiate the direct effects of alcohol.

Excessive drinking depletes the body of nutrients leading to kidney damage and cirrhosis of the liver, and ultimately to death. An often fatal complication of alcohol abuse is profoundly low blood sugar. It has been proposed that alcohol blocks gluconeogenesis by metabolic shifts that result in reduced conversions of gluconeogenic precursors into glucose and glycogen. In the absence of glycogen stores, profound hypoglycemia occurs. Hypertension may also be attributable to alcohol consumption. Three to four drinks per day causes a measurable increase in both the systolic and diastolic blood pressures. Impairments in the metabolism of vitamin A have been reported in alcoholics. Even moderate alcoholic disease is associated with severely decreased vitamin A concentrations. Riboflavin, niacin, vitamin D and vitamin E deficiency, as well as lower serum levels of ascorbic acid have been documented in alcoholics.

Alcohol also inhibits the absorption of vitamin B6 and its release from the liver. Folate deficiency is probably the most common vitamin deficiency among alcoholics. Alcohol directly inhibits enzymes involved in folate metabolism and increases urinary excretion of folate. Thiamine deficiency is observed frequently among alcoholics in whom decreased consumption and absorption and an increased requirement all appear to play a role in the development of a deficiency. Ascorbic acid has been shown to be potentially useful in alcohol detoxification. Studies of healthy men indicated that supplementation with 1 gram or 5 grams ascorbic acid daily for 2 weeks before alcohol dosing significantly enhanced the clearance of alcohol from the blood.

Caffeine

Caffeine is a derivative of xanthine. It is a pharmacologically active substance, and acts as a stimulant to the heart and central nervous system. It increases gastric acid secretion and is known to cause vasodilation. Large intakes of caffeine can induce a variety of toxic effects ranging from tremor to migraine, although as little as 200 mg can cause unpleasant effects such as sweating and palpitations. Effects are most likely when excessive quantities are taken or in highly sensitive individuals. Caffeine has an adverse effect on certain nutrients, it wastes the B vitamins and inositol. People with high blood pressure should abstain from caffeine.

Scandinavian-style boiled coffee (ground coffee beans boiled in water) was found to contain more lipid material than drip-filter coffee. Volunteers consumed a lipid-enriched fraction from boiled coffee for 6 weeks. Serum cholesterol rose in every subject. The increase was due mainly to low-density-lipoprotein cholesterol. After supplementation had ended, lipid levels returned tobaseline. Thus, boiled coffee contains a lipid that powerfully raises serum cholesterol.

Table 1

Principal food sources of caffeine

Food Caffeine	*Content*
Ground coffee (cup)	61 - 70 mg
Instant coffee (cup)	60 - 70 mg
Chocolate bar	43 - 65 mg
Carbonated cola drinks (mg/12 oz can)	15 - 75 mg
Tea (cup)	10 - 17 mg
Cocoa (cup)	97 - 125 mg

Fiber

Dietary fiber is a term used to describe a heterogeneous group of plant food components that are resistant to human digestive enzymes. It is as a non-starch polysaccharide, a type of carbohydrate. Fiber is found exclusively in plant foods. There is no RDA but we should eat at least 25 grams per day. There are two basic categories of dietary fiber:- water insoluble and water soluble. These include - cellulose, hemicellulose, gums, pectin, psyllium and lignin. Insoluble fibers are found in the skin, peel, and husks of fruit, vegetables and whole grain products. The inclusion of this fiber in a low-fat diet may reduce the risk for colon cancer. Insoluble fibers also aid in the treatment of constipation and diverticulosis.

Psyllium, oat products, barley and beans are good sources of gum, a type of soluble fiber. Gums and pectin influence absorption in the stomach and small intestine. By binding with bile acids, they decrease fat absorption and lower cholesterol levels. They coat the stomach lining, and by doing so they slow sugar absorption, regulating blood sugar levels, which is useful to diabetics since it reduces the amount of insulin needed at any one time.

Lignin also binds with bile acids, assists in lowering cholesterol levels and helps speed up food through the digestive tract. Dietary patterns emphasizing foods high in complex carbohydrates and fiber are associated with lower rates of diverticulosis, reduced risk of coronary heart disease and diabetes mellitus, lower blood glucose and blood lipid levels, and some types of cancer.

Epidemiologic evidence suggests that frequent consumption of vegetables and fruits, particularly dark green and cruciferous vegetables (such as cabbage and broccoli), may lower the risk for cancers of the lung, bladder and alimentary tract.

Whole-grain cereals, whole-grain bread, other grain bakery products and pasta, legumes - kidney beans, lima beans, navy beans, and split peas, fruits, especially the skin and edible seeds are the best source of fiber. If you think that the perilous conditions of our diet is worldwide in scope, just look at the 'underprivileged' areas of rural Africa. In the year 1975, the southern areas of rural Africa avoided the major scourges of the modern world. British doctors found in their research on rural African villages that cancer of the colon and the rectum is extremely rare, and that there is no appendicitis, hemorrhoids, obesity, heart attacks, varicose veins, phlebitis, or diverticulosis of the colon. As if this evidence were not enough proof that something is wrong with our diet, it has been shown that Africans develop the same diseases we have as soon as they adopt a Western diet-that is, as soon as they cut their intake of roughage.

Gelatin

The most notable characteristic of gelatin is that it is soluble in hot water but forms a solid jelly when it cools. The Latin word gelatus means frozen, and is recalled in the Italian word for ice cream, gelati. Gelatin is a protein, and is formed from collagen, which is the primary protein in connective tissue. Animal bones, skin and gristly meat are a major source of gelatin. By itself gelatin has a low biological value. Commercial jellies with their sugar and flavour make an attractive desert, but with their 2% of an inferior protein, it is unrealistic to suppose that because they are solid they add significantly to the nourishment of a convalescent.

Agar is a vegetable gelling agent, and since, unlike gelatin it is not derived from an animal source it is used as an alternative to gelatin, by vegetarians and people following a kosher diet, in many of the same foods.

Gluten

Gluten is a mixture of two proteins, gliadin and glutenin. It is the presence of gluten in wheat and rye that makes these cerealssuitable for the production of bread. When mixed with water and kneaded, the gluten in wheat or rye flour becomes elastic and traps small bubbles of carbon dioxide from yeast fermentation. The flour of other cereals such as oats or maize, with little or no gluten, can be used only for flat cakes such as tortillas. Children with coeliac disease, and some adults with a similar disease known as sprue, have a sensitivity to gluten which causes damage to the intestinal villi so that they are unable to properly digest and absorb some of the food components, especially fat. It has been suggested that several other unrelated diseases, including schizophrenia and multiple sclerosis, in some patients may be caused by a sensitivity to gluten. The evidence for these claims is not conclusive and has not been substantiated.

Nevertheless, it does seem as if some babies without obvious coeliac disease are sensitive to gluten although they lose this sensitivity gradually through their first few months or years. For this reason many manufacturers of baby foods avoid using gluten-containing items in their products.

Lecithin

Lecithin is a phosphatide or phospholipid, a fatty substance found in animal and plant tissues. It is composed of choline, phosphoric acid, two fatty acids and glycerol. Lecithin is produced by the liver and passes into the intestine, to be absorbed into the blood. As an emulsifying agent it allows fats and cholesterol to flow easily in the blood stream and through arterial walls.

It is essential in maintaining the surface tension of cell membranes, and in controlling cellular intake and secretion. It also helps in conducting impulses to and from nerve cells. It has also been shown to control heart disease and atherosclerosis. If enough lecithin is present the disease does not occur. The best natural sources of lecithin are eggs, wheat, soya oil and nuts. It is also readily available in supplement form.

Monosodium Glutamite (MSG)

MSG, usually manufactured from wheat gluten, is used not because of its own flavour but because it enhances the flavour of stews, soups, savoury sauces and cooked vegetables. MSG is the sodium salt of glutamic acid, an amino acid found in most proteins and thus present in the gravies of cooked meats and protein derivatives such as hydrolyzed vegetable protein. MSG is found in many Chinese foods, partly because it is present in soya sauce and because the pure substance is often used. It is also found in dried soups and many other prepared foods. Some individuals react to MSG by what is called the Chinese Restaurant Syndrome. This is characterized by pain in the neck, headache and perhaps palpitations. This condition is only transitory and individuals sensitive to MSG soon learn to avoid eating foods containing it.

Oxalic Acid (Oxalate)

In the small amounts normally present in food, the only importance of oxalic acid is that it combines with calcium in the diet and so reduces the amount of this mineral element that can be absorbed. Large quantities may cause poisoning by damaging the lining of the mouth and stomach, and interfering with the action of the nerves and muscles. A few foods, notably unripe tomatoes and some varieties of strawberries, may have small amounts. However, beetroot has about 100 milligrams per 100 grams, parsley about 150 milligrams, and rhubarb and spinach between 300 and 600 milligrams. As well as deriving oxalate from the diet, the body can synthesize it from citric acid. Some urinary stones contain calcium oxalate, as well as other calcium salts, but it is not known to what extent this is derived from dietary oxalic acid or from excessive synthesis.

Nevertheless, if a person is known to excrete an excessive amount of oxalate in the urine, or to have had kidney stones containing oxalate, it is reasonable to restrict the consumption of spinach and rhubarb, as well as chocolate and cocoa.

Phytic Acid (Phytate)

Phytic acid is a compound of inositol and phosphoric acid. It occurs partly as an acid and partly as salts such as calcium phytate in plant foods, especially in the bran of cereals, and in pulses and nuts. It readily combines with minerals including calcium, iron and zinc, and if these are present in only marginally adequate amounts in the diet, phytic acid may reduce their availability sufficiently to cause deficiency. There are, however, a few ways in which this hazard is reduced.

Germination, soaking fermentation and cooking all reduce the effect of phytate in legumes. Flour has calcium carbonate added to it in amounts more than enough for all the phytic acid present to be converted to the insoluble calcium phytate. The yeast used for providing dough contains an enzyme, phytase, that breaks down much of the phytic acid. The body gradually adapts to much of thephytic acid in the diet, perhaps by an increase in the amount phytase in the intestine, so that after time its effect in reducing the availability of calcium and other elements diminishes.

Psyllium (Plantago ovata)

Psyllium is obtained from the seed husks of a plant grown in India and the Mediterranean region. It contains eight times the soluble fiber of oat bran. When included as a part of a low-fat, low-cholesterol, high-fiber diet, psyllium has been found to be effective in lowering blood cholesterol levels, especially LDL-cholesterol. Since 1930, the primary use of psyllium has been a bulk forming laxative. Approximately four million people in the United States use a commercial pharmaceutical form of psyllium. The acute toxicity of psyllium is very low. In 1981, a committee of the National Research Council concluded that "There is no evidence in the available information on psyllium husk gum that demonstrates or suggests reasonable grounds to suspect a hazard to the public when it is used at levels that are now current or that might reasonably be expected in the future."

Steroids

Steroids are a group of organic compounds including sterols, of which the best known is cholesterol. It has received attention in conection with circulatory ailments, especially hardening of the arteries. If excess cholesterol is present in the body, it tends to precipitate from solution in the gall bladder as gallstones, and in the blood vessels where the constriction thus formed reduces blood flow, causing high blood pressure. Other sterols produced in the ovaries and testes, that control the physiology of the reproductive process and the secondary sex characteristics, are known as sex hormones. Although primarily involved with reproductive mechanisims, sex hormones are also significant as growth substances of general importance to body health and well-being.

The female sex hormones, the estrogens are essential for the changes of the menstrual cycle, and progesterone which prepares the uterus for fertilization and is required for normal pregnancy. Progesterone, now produced synthetically, is used clinically to prevent abortion in certain difficult pregnancies. The male sex hormones, androgens, regulate the development of reproductive organs and secondary sex characteristics such as beards, deep voices, etc.

Some steroids that are synthesized commercially are used for muscle and bone growth in athletes and body builders. The abuse of anabolic-androgenic steroids has been well documented in bodybuilders, and the potential for harmful side effects clearly exposed. Adverse reactions may include increased risks of the following: liver diseases, including liver cancer, heart disease and stroke, decreased immune function, acquired immune deficiency syndrome (AIDS), kidney stones and diseases, gall stones, hypertension, prostate enlargement, testicular atrophy, sterility, impotence, stunted growth in adolescents, psychological changes, irreversible virilization in women, and fetal damage.

The well documented negative effects far outweigh the short term benefits of steroid usage. There is no long term advantage of using steroids as ultimately they are going to cause harm to your system.

Tannins

Tannins are one of the phenolic compounds (phenolic acid, coumarins, flavonoids) that are widely distributed in plants, conferring increased resistance to pests. Tannin effects in human beings range from pharmacologic, therapeutic, and aesthetic benefits to anti-nutritional and other undesirable results. Plant tannins can complex with and precipitate proteins. Sorghum tannin can bind up to 12 times its weight in protein. Condensed tannins, the major phenols in commonly consumed foods and beverages such as fruit, vegetables, tea, red wine, cocoa, legumes, certain grains (sorghum, millet), and pulses, are more nutritionally hazardous. Concern for potential nutritional hazards, therefore, is for populations that rely on sorghum, millet, or certain legumes as their dietary staple.

Decreases in growth rate, feeding efficiency, and protein digestibility are some of the effects caused by complexing of phenols with protein, starch, digestive enzymes, vitamins and minerals. Additionally, malnutrition enhances tannin toxicity. Attempts to inactivate or remove tannins from foods and feeds have had limited results.

Tartrazine

Tartrazine is used in foods, beverages, drugs and cosmetics. It has been estimated that about 100 000 persons in the United States are sensitive to this substance. Symptoms of allergy include generalized urticaria, swelling, often of the face and lips, runny nose, and on occasion even life threatening asthma. Since tartrazine is found in a large number of products,tartrazine-sensitive individuals are advised to read labels and avoid food containing "FD&C Yellow No. 5".

Water

Although water is often excluded from lists of nutrients, it is an essential dietary component, in that it must be acquired from the diet in amounts well in excess of that produced by metabolism in the body. Water is the most abundant constituent of the human body, accounting for about four-fifths of body weight.

Waste products need to be excreted from the body. This process of excretion is done by the kidneys, where the nitrogen-containing products of protein metabolism, sulfates, phosphates and other electrolytes are dissolved in water and excreted as urine. To compensate for this loss, a thirst sensation is created. If this thirst sensation is not met with an adequate consumption of water, dehydration will occur. Toxicity results from the ingestion of water at a rate beyond the capacity of the kidneys to excrete it. The manifestations usually include a gradual mental dulling, confusion, convulsion, coma and death.

Recommended Dietary Allowances

Food and Nutrition Board, National Academy of Sciences - Recommended Dietary Allowances, Revised 1989

Designed for the maintenance of good nutrition of practically all healthy people in the United States. The allowances, expressed as average daily intakes over time, are intended to provide for individual variations among most normal persons as they live in the United States under usual environmental stresses. Diets should be based on a variety of common foods in order to provide other nutrients for which human requirements have been less well defined. See text for detailed discussion of allowances and of nutrients not tabulated.

Because there are uncertainties in the knowledge base, it is not possible to set RDAs for all the known nutrients. However, the RDAs can serve as a guide such that a varied diet meeting RDAs will probably be adequate in all other nutrients. Therefore, the subcommittee recommends that diets should be composed of a variety of foods that are derived from diverse food groups rather than by supplementation or fortification and that losses of nutrients during the processing and preparation of food should be taken into consideration in planning diets.

RDAs apply to healthy persons. They do not cover special nutritional needs arising from metabolic disorders, chronic diseases, injuries, premature birth, other medical conditions, and drug therapies.

*Weights and heights of Reference Adults are actual medians for the U.S. population of the designated age, as reported by NHANES II. The use of these figures does not imply that the height-to-weight ratios are ideal.

Table 2

Weight, Height, Protein requirement

Category	*Age (Years)*	*Weight (Kg)*	*Height (cm)*	*Protein (g)*
Infants	0 - ½	6	60	13
Infants	½ - 1	9	71	14
Children	1 - 3	13	90	16
Children	4 - 6	20	112	24
Children	7 - 10	28	132	28
Males	11 - 14	45	157	45
Males	15 - 18	66	176	59
Males	19 - 24	72	177	58
Males	25 - 50	79	176	63
Males	51 +	77	173	63
Females	11 - 14	46	157	46
Females	15 - 18	55	163	44
Females	19 - 24	58	164	46
Females	25 - 50	63	163	50
Females	51 +	65	160	50

Diet Planning

The fact that more than 20% of the United States adult population is obese presents a major public health concern. However, the failure to follow through and maintain weight loss on their own, after termination of counselling, makes the long-term success of weight loss programs difficult to achieve. Health professionals often assume that patients will dutifully comply with recommendations simply because they are urged to do so.

The magnitude of noncompliance has been well documented. Adherence to dietary programs is thought to be poorer than to medication regimens. Dietary regimens are often restrictive, require changes in life-style and behaviours, interfere with family habits and customs, and are of long duration.

Weight control methods are considered a success if weight loss is maintained without expense to overall health. A goal of any successful weight reduction program is to promote permanent life-style changes. The physical and psychological consequences of repeated weight fluctuations may be more harmful than maintaining some degree of overweight. The ultimate goal of all weight loss programs is to reduce nutritional risk factors associated with chronic diseases by increasing consumer awareness of healthy food choices.

In 1992 over 49 million people were dieting. The National Council Against Fraud estimates that quackery costs consumers between $25 billion and $50 billion a year - and nutrition fraud is the most common type. Therefore to identify a quality weight loss program, and not to be misled by a "fad diet", the following indicators must be considered:

— *A variety of foods:* Weight control programs should be individualized to fit people's life-styles and food preferences. Individualization diminishes feelings of deprivation, which lead to discouragement, bingeing, and rebound weight gain - all hallmarks of the yo-yo diet syndrome.

— *Enough calories to maintain good health:* Consuming less than 1200 kcal a day may result in loss of muscle instead of fat and may compromise nutritional status as a result of deficient nutrient intakes.

— *Realistic weight loss goals:* To lose body fat and not just water, a maximum weight loss of 2 pounds per week is advised.

— *Regular exercise:* Especially as we age, exercise can be the key to weight loss and maintenance of a desirable weight.

— *Behaviour modification:* Registered dietitians counsel people to keep lost weight off by helping them alter their eating behavior and responses to foods for the rest of their lives.

Unfortunately, a current trend toward the view that a single food is either a panacea or a poison is being gradually adopted by major health associations. This "good food/bad food" dichotomy ignores the consensus among nutritionists that all foods can be compatible with health when used in moderation as part of a balanced, varied diet. Over the past decade people have become obsessed with the nutritional value of the food they eat. Time and again, nutrition ranks high among consumer concerns, along with food safety, convenience, quality, and value. In the United States sales in the "healthy foods" category accounted for $65 billion in 1985, but are expected to reach $98 billion by 1995.

Consumers are asking for specific information about which foods and, in particular, which brands of packaged foods to choose from when they eat or purchase foods. For example the broad guideline to avoid to much fat, saturated fat and cholesterol require specific behaviour implementations that include:

Eat more fresh fruits and vegetables, whole grain breads and cereals, potatoes, rice noodles, dried beans, peas, and lentils. Choose low fat dairy products, including skim, 1%, and 2% milk, low-fat cheeses, and low-fat yogurt. Choose lean meats, fish, chicken and turkey.

Diet and Nutrition

This section is concerned with the nutritional requirements for the healthy person, and for the sick, wounded, and convalescing patient. Research has confirmed that good health depends in part upon the availability of essential nutrients the body requires throughout life. The well-nourished individual is usually mentally alert, is at a maximum of physical capability, and has a high resistance to disease.

The daily basic minimum nutritional requirements must be met and often supplemented during periods of illness to meet the changing needs of the body and its ability to use foods. Therefore, the diet is an important factor in the therapeutic plan for each patient.

The important role of nutrition in overall health is widely recognized. As a member of the Navy, you must be healthy to perform your professional duties. Part of maintaining a healthy lifestyle starts with eating a well-balanced diet and maintaining a good fitness regimen. Many people in the Navy and Marine Corps do not maintain a proper daily diet. As a Hospital Corpsman, you may be responsible for providing nutritional counseling and, perhaps, even motivation. You have an added responsibility to observe for additional nutritional needs and omissions and to advise your shipmates when necessary. If you stay healthy and energetic, the knowledge and experience you share and the example you set may help your shipmates adopt and maintain a healthier lifestyle.

Balancing energy intake and expenditure can be difficult, both when activity levels are high as well as when they are very low. Typically, body weight remains constant when energy intake equals expenditure. The energy balance equation can be 'unbalanced' by changing energy intake, energy expenditure, or both. To gain or lose 1 pound requires that approximately 3,500 extra calories be consumed or burned.

Food Classification

Foods are substances from animal and plant sources that yield heat and energy when ingested and absorbed by the body. Food nutrients build and renew tissues and regulate the body processes. The unit commonly used for describing energy intake and energy expenditure is the calorie. Good food sources contain substantial amounts of nutrients in relation to caloric content and provide upwards of 10 percent of the U.S. Recommended Dietary Allowance for each specific nutrient.

Most people can get enough of each required nutrient daily by eating a wide variety of foods.

Proteins

Proteins are the 'building blocks' of the body and provide important required nutritive elements. Proteins are needed for growth, maintenance, and replacement of body cells, and they form hormones and enzymes used to regulate body processes. Extra protein is either used to supply energy or is changed into body fat. Found in both the animal and plant kingdoms, all proteins are composed of amino acids.

Some amino acids are absolutely essential to maintain life and are necessary for repair, growth, and body development. Of the approximately 20 amino acids, our body can produce all but nine. These nine amino acids are termed 'essential amino acids.' We must get them from food, and we need all nine at one time so our body can use them effectively.

Proteins, which promote tissue growth and renewal, have long been recognized as the main structural unit of all living cells. Each gram (g) of protein yields 4 calories in the process of metabolism. Although proteins yield energy, they are an expensive source. If sufficient carbohydrates are not supplied, the body will use protein for energy requirements. This protein may be obtained from muscle tissue, producing the 'wasting effect' of long-term starvation and some diseases.

A constant protein source is required in the daily diet. The normal daily protein intake for adults should be 0.8 gram per kilogram (g/kg) (2.2 lbs) of body weight, or 12 percent of the total caloric intake. Pregnant women require an additional 10 grams of protein a day over the normal daily intake. Proteins play an important role in recovering from fractures, burns, and infections. They are also important in healing wounds and recovering from surgical procedures. In cases of recovery, protein intake should be increased in accordance with the severity of the condition, and carbohydrates and fats can be added liberally. While proteins can supply energy, they are not a main source of energy like carbohydrates and fat.

Ideally, the patient should receive protein by mouth; however, it is sometimes necessary to meet the minimum requirements parenterally. Glucose parenteral solution, given during an acute emergency period, will prevent some loss of protein. Protein deficiency may stunt growth, promote a secondary anemia, or induce nutritional edema. Dietary sources of protein and the nine essential amino acids are milk, yogurt, eggs, meats, fish, cheese, poultry, peanut butter, legumes, and nuts. Protein from plant sources is best when combined with animal protein, such as milk plus peanut butter, or when legumes are combined with grains, such as Navy beans plus rice.

Fats

The chief functions of fats are to supply energy and transport fat-soluble vitamins. Each gram of fat yields 9 calories. Fats provide the most concentrated source of calories (and, therefore, energy) of all the food nutrients. Fats are found in both the animal and vegetable kingdoms. Fatty acids and glycerol are the end products of the digestion of fats. Many fats act as carriers for the fat-soluble vitamins A, D, E, and K. They also act both as a padding for vital organs, particularly the kidneys, and as subcutaneous tissue to help conserve body heat. Fat is stored as adipose (fatty) tissue to form a reserve supply in time of need.

Dietary fats delay gastric emptying and promote a feeling of fullness. Excess calories from fats may produce obesity, the forerunner of arteriosclerosis, hypertension, gallbladder disease, and diabetes. Adiet high in fat, especially saturated fat and cholesterol, contributes to elevated blood cholesterol levels in many people. Adults over the age of 30 should have a serum cholesterol level of less than 200 mg/dl. Health experts agree that less than 30 percent of our total calories per day should come from fat. Saturated fat intake should be no more than 10 percent of the total calories.

Reducing dietary fat is also a good way to limit calories. Decreased fat intake results in fewer calories without a reduction of most nutrients. Too little fat in the diet may lead to being underweight, having insufficient padding for the vital organs, and lowered energy. Butter, margarine, cream cheese, fatty meats, whole milk, olives, avocados, egg yolks, nuts, commercial bakery products, and vegetable oils are all sources of dietary fat.

Carbohydrates (sugar and starches) are the most efficient sources of energy and are known as the 'fuel of life. They are abundantly found in most plant food sources. Complex carbohydrates (starches) are in breads, cereals, pasta, rice, dry beans and peas, and other vegetables, such as potatoes and corn. Simple carbohydrates are found in sugars, honey, syrup, jam, and many desserts. The new nutritional guidelines established by the Food and Drug Administration (FDA) recommend that complex carbohydrates and naturally occurring sugars (found primarily in fruit) make up approximately 50 percent of one's total caloric intake. The FDA also recommends that refined and processed sugars make up no more than 10 percent of the calories in one's diet.

Each gram of carbohydrate yields 4 calories in the process of its metabolism. Carbohydrates must be reduced to glucose before the body can use them. Carbohydrates are stored in the muscles to fuel their movement, and in the liver as glycogen, which is then broken down and released as glucose at the exact rate needed by the body. This latter mechanism is controlled largely by insulin from the pancreas. During fasting, liver glycogen is rapidly depleted, leading the body to use its fat for energy. Carbohydrates that are not needed for energy are converted to and stored as adipose (fat) tissue. The main functions of carbohydrates are to

— furnish the main source of energy for muscular work and nutritive processes,

— help maintain body temperature,

— form reserve fuel,

— assist in oxidation of fats, and

— spare protein for growth and repair.

Vitamin and Mineral Supplements

Vitamin supplements are usually not necessary if a diet includes a wide variety of foods. Exceptions may occur in prenatal diets in which iron is low, as well as in patients who are deficient in a specific vitamin. Vitamin supplements should be taken only on a physician or dietitian's recommendation. Vitamin and mineral supplements are being widely used by physically active people because of all the performance-enhancing claims made by supplement manufacturers. It is estimated that 40-50 percent of athletes use some form of vitamin/mineral supplements. Some doses range from amounts similar to the Recommended Dietary Allowances (RDA) up to levels many times the RDA. Supplements are useful under a variety of conditions, such as if an individual

— has an existing vitamin or mineral deficiency;

— has poor nutrient intake and/or dietary habits; or

— is exposed to extreme environmental conditions, such as altitude.

Often, laxatives are prescribed in conjunction with some medical treatments and may cause decreased absorption of vitamins, loss of minerals and electrolytes, or inhibition of glucose uptake. Therefore, any patient on laxatives should be carefully monitored, and supplementary nutritives should be administered as necessary. Taking a general multivitamin supplement appears to be without measurable performance enhancing effects in healthy, well-nourished, physically active personnel. Similarly, no improvements in muscle strength or endurance have been noted in strength athletes, such as body builders, who tend to use megadoses of vitamin and mineral supplements. The indiscriminate use of high-potency vitamins and minerals is of growing concern since excessive amounts of vitamins and/or minerals can be harmful and may result in nutrient imbalances. Excessive intake of some vitamin and mineral supplements can result in adverse and possibly toxic side effects.

The Food Guide Pyramid

The Food Guide Pyramid emphasizes foods from the five food groups shown in the sections of the pyramid. Each of these groups provides some, but not all, of the nutrients we require. For good health we need them all. For everyday living, the simplest and most practical plan is to follow those same guidelines, selecting from the various food groups the type and amount of food recommended.

Dietary Guidelines

The food pyramid graphically communicates the message of the Dietary Guidelines for Americans. Diets should be built upon a base of complex carbohydrates and less fats. The placement of the food groups starting at the base of the pyramid conveys the current recommendations. These recommendations are as follows:

— Eat more grains, vegetables, and fruits

— Eat moderate amounts of lean meats and dairy foods

— Use sweets, fats, and oils sparingly

Generally accepted guidelines suggest that you eat a diet that is high in complex carbohydrates and low in protein and fat. Your diet should consist of at least five combined servings of fruits and vegetables each day. Avoid fat when possible. Eat at regular intervals when possible, and avoid snacking late at night.

Diet Therapy

It is often necessary to cater to a patient's appetite, since many individuals become especially hard to please when sick. In some disease states, such as cancer, patients experience marked taste changes. Because of the importance of the nutritional elements in feeding the sick, try to carry out the patient's wishes whenever possible. A tactful and observant

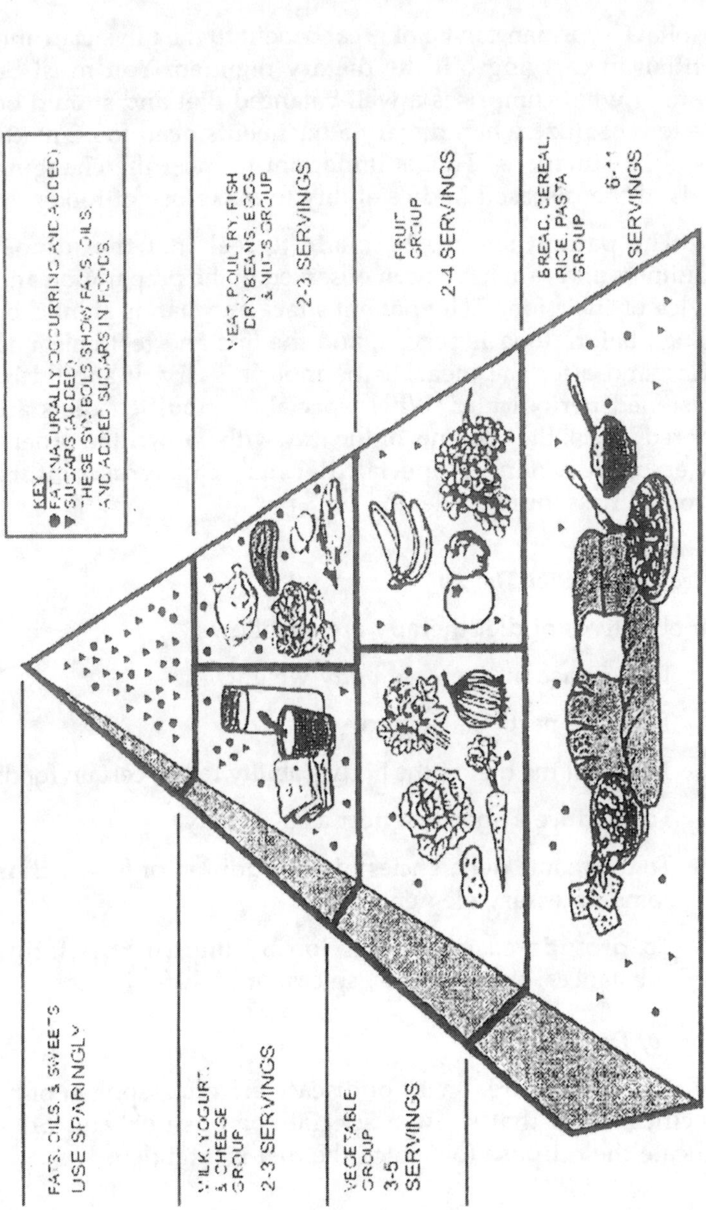

Figure 1. Food Guide Pyramid.

Hospital Corpsman can be of great benefit to the physician and dietitian in carrying out the dietary regimen. You must be aware of what comprises a well-balanced diet and should be able to recognize when dietary adjustments need to be made in special situations. This is important to meet the changing needs of the diseased body's ability to make use of foods.

The patient should be made to feel that the utmost cleanliness and care have been observed in the preparation and service of their food. The patient's face and hands should be cleaned before food is served, and the lips and teeth cleaned before and after the meal. If the mouth is dry, it should be moistened periodically. When special or modified diets are ordered, check the contents of the tray with the written orders. An error in serving a special diet may cause discomfort, serious illness, or even death.

Objectives of Diet Therapy

The objectives of diet therapy are as follows:

- To increase or decrease body weight
- To rest a particular organ
- To adjust the diet to the body's ability to use certain foods
- To produce a specific effect as a remedy
- To overcome deficiencies by the addition of food rich in some necessary element
- To provide ease of digestion by omitting irritating substances, such as fiber, spices, or high-fat foods

Types of Diets

Diets used in the treatment of disease are often spoken of by specific names that show a special composition and often indicate the purpose for which the diet is intended.

Regular Diet

The regular diet is composed of all types of foods and is well balanced and capable of maintaining a state of good nutrition. It is intended for convalescing patients who do not require a therapeutic diet.

Modified or Therapeutic Diets

Modified or therapeutic diets are modifications of the regular diet and are designed to meet specific patient needs. These include

— method of preparation (e.g., baking, boiling, or broiling),

— consistency (e.g., ground or chopped),

— total calories (e.g., high or low calorie),

— nutrients (e.g., altering carbohydrate, protein, fat, vitamins, and minerals), and

— allowing only specific foods (e.g., diabetic diet).

Soft diet

The soft diet is soft in texture and consists of liquids and semi-solid foods. It is indicated in certain postoperative cases, for convalescents who cannot tolerate a regular diet, in acute illnesses, and in some gastrointestinal disorders. A soft diet is an intermediate step between a liquid and regular diet and is low in connective tissue and indigestible dietary fiber. Little or no spices are used in its preparation.

The soft diet includes all liquids other than alcohol, and foods that may be incorporated into a soft diet include well-cooked cereals, pastas, white bread and crackers, eggs, cottage cheese, tender meat, fish, poultry, and vegetables (including baked, mashed, and scalloped potatoes).

Vegetables can be purred and meats ground for dental patients. Permitted desserts are custards, gelatin puddings, soft fruits, and simple cakes and cookies. Foods prohibited in a soft diet include fried foods, raw vegetables, and nuts.

Liquid Diet

A liquid diet consists of foods that are in a liquid state at body temperature. This type of diet is indicated in some postoperative cases, in acute illnesses, and in inflammatory conditions of the gastrointestinal (GI) tract. It is important that feedings consisting of 6 to 8 ounces or more be given every 2 to 3 hours while the patient is awake.

Liquid diets are usually ordered as clear, full, or dental liquid. A clear liquid diet includes clear broth, black tea or coffee, plain gelatin, and clear fruit juices (apple, grape, and cranberry), popsicles, fruit drinks, and soft drinks. This diet is inadequate in all nutrients. A full liquid diet includes all the liquids served on a clear liquid diet, with the addition of strained cream soups, milk and milk drinks, ice cream, puddings, and custard. The full liquid diet is inadequate in iron, niacin, and possibly Vitamin A and thiamin. A dental liquid diet includes regular foods blended and strained in liquid form and all foods allowed on clear and full liquid diets. Vitamin and mineral supplements may be necessary with the dental liquid diet if the recommended amounts of food are not tolerated.

High Calorie Diet

The high-calorie diet is of a higher caloric value than the average patient normally requires. A high-calorie diet is indicated when an increase of total calories is required by malnourished, underweight, post surgical, or convalescing patients, especially those recovering from acute illnesses such as infections, burns, and fevers. The increase in calories is obtained by supplementing or modifying the regular diet with high-calorie foods or commercial supplements, by giving larger portions, or by adding snacks. It is given to meet a need for energy caused by the more rapid metabolism that accompanies certain diseases.

In the liquid or soft diet, adding fats and carbohydrates increases the caloric value. The high-calorie diet is often ordered along with high protein. Proteins are added to prevent depletion of proteins in the plasma (a condition known as hypoproteinemia). As the patient progresses, a more solid diet is given.

Good sources of high-calorie foods are whole milk, cream, sweets, butter, margarine, fried foods, gravy, sauces, and ice cream. Between-meal feedings consisting of milk, milkshakes, cheese, cookies, or sandwiches are recommended, but these feedings should not interfere with the patient's appetite at mealtime.

High-Protein Diet

As previously stated, protein is essential for tissue growth and regeneration. A high-protein diet is indicated in almost all illnesses (e.g., nephrosis, cirrhosis of the liver, infectious hepatitis, burns, radiation injury, fractures, so. GI disorders, conditions in which the protein blood level is low, and in preoperative and postoperative cases). In some acute illnesses and disorders, such as infectious hepatitis, GI disorders, and postoperative conditions, patients may be unable to consume solid foods or the daily requirement of protein and calories because of pain or nausea.

In these cases, intravenous fluids with nutrient additives are required for the patient to receive the required amount of protein. Protein-calorie deficiency is a definite factor in postoperative wound disruption. This disruption can best be prevented by preemptive nutritional measures before surgery. Antibody production will be decreased if the patient receives inadequate protein. Remember, the daily recommended intake of proteins for adults is at least 0.8 g/kg of body weight (approximately 56 g).

Ahigh-protein diet should provide a minimum of 1.5 g of protein per kg of body weight (approximately 105 g). The seriously burned and radiation injury patients should receive at least 3.0 g/kg daily. Supplement the regular diet with high-quality protein foods, such as meat, fish, cheese, milk, and eggs.

Low-Calorie Diet

The low-calorie diet is useful in the treatment of obesity, but it may also be used to control weight in medical conditions such as arthritis, hypertension, diabetes, cardiac disease, or hypothyroidism. A loss of 1 to 2 pounds per week is the medically acceptable limit for weight reduction. A low-calorie diet consists of 1,000 to 1,800 calories per day. Calorie levels are determined by physicians and dietitians to help meet specific individual patient weight-loss goals. The daily intake of proteins should be at least 0.8 g/kg of standard body weight. Supplemental vitamins may be ordered if the prescribed diet is less than 1,200 calories. Patients on low-calorie diets should be instructed by the dietitian or other medical personnel knowledgeable in proper eating habits.

The dietitian conducts patient interviews to learn the patient's eating behaviors, usual portions, preparation of foods, meal patterns, nutritional adequacy, exercise, and so forth. Individual programs should then be recommended to assist patients to attain and maintain their ideal weight.

The Handbook of Clinical Dietetics, published by the American Dietetic Association, lists the following formula for determining ideal body weight. For females, the basic weight for 5 feet is 100 pounds. Add 5 pounds for every inch over 5 feet. For males, the basic weight for 5 feet is 106 pounds, with 6 pounds added for every inch over 5 feet. Adjustments must be made for body build. Reduce desired weight by 10 percent for a small frame; increase it by 10 percent for a large frame. Total caloric requirements are based on ideal body weight plus activity.

Many patients on low-calorie diets experience hunger. To satisfy this hunger or appetite, low-calorie foods such as raw vegetables, broth, black coffee or tea, and other unsweetened or diet beverages should be provided. Water and sodium need not be restricted unless there are cardiac complications or edema, and the restrictions are ordered by the physician.

Low Protein Diet

As the name implies, the low-protein diet is made up of foods that furnish only small amounts of protein and consist largely of carbohydrates and fats (e.g., foods such as marshmallows, hard candy, and butter). This diet is used in renal diseases associated with nitrogen retention or liver disorders. Limited amounts of protein are sometimes advocated in certain kidney diseases (such as chronic nephrotic edema). Low-protein diets for renal failure are usually restricted in sodium and potassium, because these two elements are not excreted properly during this condition. In some cases of chronic renal insufficiency, the protein content of the diet is varied, usually between 40 and 60 g per day, so that there will be sufficient complete protein to maintain nitrogen equilibrium. In some metabolic disturbances, such as amino acids in the urine, protein restriction may be of therapeutic value.

High-Residue Diet

The high-residue (high-bulk, high-fiber, high-roughage) diet is indicated in atonic constipation, spastic colon, irritable bowel syndrome, and diverticulosis. This diet encourages regular elimination by stimulating muscle tone, creating softer and larger stools that are more easily propelled through the colon, thereby reducing the pain and cramping that accompany spastic colon or irritable bowel syndrome.

The patient is given a regular diet, with the inclusion of high-residue foods. The main sources of fiber are whole-grain breads and cereals, bran cereals, fresh fruits, and vegetables that are raw or cooked until tender. Whole grain breads and cereals that contain wheat bran have a greater laxative effect than fruits and vegetables, because the bran acts to absorb water within the colon, creating a bulk effect. Fiber intake should be increased gradually to minimize potential side effects of bloating, cramps, and diarrhea.

At least one serving of 100 percent wheat bran cereal is recommended daily. Cereals such as raisin bran, Bran Flakes',

Shredded Wheat', and oatmeal may be used occasionally, but they contain less than half the amount of fiber found in All-Bran, or Bran Buds. Fresh fruits and vegetables with edible skins, such as apples and grapes, are higher in fiber content than canned fruits or vegetables and their juices.

Dietary intake of refined sugars and starches should be decreased because they are poor sources of fiber. Also, limit white flour products, refined cereals, pies, cakes, and cookies. Too little fluid in the high-residue diet may cause dehydration and lead to constipation. The patient must drink at least eight 8-ounce glasses of water or other fluids daily, particularly when consuming the recommended amount of bran. Drinking too much alcohol, beverages containing caffeine (such as coffee, cola, tea, and soft drinks), however, can irritate a sensitive colon and can cause dehydration. When possible, use decaffeinated coffee.

One or two glasses of water in the morning help to stimulate peristalsis. Excessive intake of foods like dried beans, fruits with seeds and skins, nuts, popcorn, and strong spices may cause irritability, especially during the inflammation period of colon disease states. These foods should be individualized to the patient. When one is progressing from a low-residue diet after an acute infection or diverticulitis, increase fiber in the diet gradually. Start by adding one serving of 100 percent bran cereal and three servings of whole-grain bread to the low-residue menu pattern. Gradually increase the amount of raw vegetables and fresh fruits to at least four servings per day.

Low Residue Diet

The low-residue diet is indicated in ulceration, inflammation, and other gastric disorders. It is also used in certain postoperative states that affect any part of the GI tract, e.g., a hemorrhoidectomy. Low-residue diets are also used in treating dysenteries of long duration. The purpose of this diet is to provide nonstimulating, non-irritating, and easily digested material that leaves little residue, thus avoiding mechanical irritation of the GI tract. Various commercially prepared low-residue elemental diet supplements may be given to provide complete nutrition.

Low Sodium Diet

A low-sodium diet consists of foods containing a very small percentage of sodium, with no salt added in preparation or by the patient. It is impossible to prepare an absolutely sodium-free diet.

The low-sodium diet is indicated when edema is present, in renal diseases, hypertension, and certain cardiac conditions. The nephrotic patient is often unable to excrete sodium in a normal manner because the kidneys' retention of sodium leads to edema. A low-sodium diet is thus indicated, with no restriction on salt-free liquids. Such patients should be encouraged to drink 2,000 to 3,000 milliliters (ml) of low-sodium fluids daily.

The allowance of sodium in a strict low-sodium diet is 250 to 1,000 mg daily. The allowance of sodium in a moderate low-sodium diet is 2,000 mg or 2 g. Regular diets with no salt added contain 2.4 to 4.5 g of sodium.

Any diet in which the amount of sodium is drastically reduced has possible side effects. The patient who is on this diet regimen must be constantly observed-particularly in warm climates-for lassitude, complaints of weakness, anorexia, nausea and vomiting, mental confusion, abdominal cramps, and aching skeletal muscles. Electrolyte imbalances can have serious consequences. If you observe symptoms such as those described above, notify a medical officer.

Bland Diet

A bland diet may be helpful for gastritis, hyperacidity, hemorrhoids, peptic ulcers, and other GI disorders. Dietary management of patients with chronic ulcer disease has been the subject of much controversy. Bland diets have traditionally been used for these patients. However, experiments show that there is no significant difference in the response of patients with an active duodenal ulcer to a bland diet. Known irritants to the gastric mucosa include alcohol, black pepper, caffeine, chili powder, cocoa, coffee, certain drugs, and tea.

Emphasizing how to eat is as important as indicating what foods to eat, since there are individual responses to bland diets. Offer the following suggestions to the patient:

— Avoid worry and emotional upsets at mealtime

— Chew food well and eat slowly

— Rest before and after meals

— Avoid foods of extreme temperatures

If fruits and juices between meals cause distress, try including them with meals. Meals must be kept small to reduce gastric acidity and distention. Among foods to avoid in the bland diet are

— fatty meats,

— fried foods,

— whole-grain breads and cereals,

— dried beans and peas,

— cabbage-family vegetables,

— chocolate,

— nuts and seeds, and

— carbonated beverages, caffeine, coffee, and tea.

Patients on a bland diet may use spices and condiments such as allspice, cinnamon, mace, paprika, sage, thyme, catsup, cranberry or mint jelly, and extract and flavorings without chocolate or vinegar. The bland diet allows a more liberal food selection than other restrictive diets. This diet reduces the number of meals to three, and increases the quantity of foods given. Individualize the diet to the patient. The 'Regular-No

Stimulants Diet' (also called ìliberal bland'), a type of bland diet, eliminates only those items that have been shown scientifically to irritate the gastric mucosa (i.e., alcohol, black pepper, caffeine, chili powder, cocoa, coffee, certain drugs, and tea).

Decaffeinated coffee may be restricted in most types of bland diets. Recent studies show that it causes increased gastric acid secretion and esophageal pressure causing gastric acid reflux in the esophagus. Decaffeinated coffee is only offered on the bland diet and the regular-no stimulants diet if it is tolerated by the patient. Chronic and excessive use of antacids to treat hyperacidity and related conditions may result in thiamin deficiency, presumably because of alkaline destruction of thiamin within the bowel lumen. Excessive intake of milk with antacids may cause systemic alkalosis and hypercalcemia. Milk may be contraindicated in patients with allergic reactions or lactose intolerance.

Low-Carbohydrate, High Protein diet

A low-carbohydrate, high-protein diet is used in the treatment of hypoglycemia. This diet limits simple carbohydrates that are quickly absorbed into the blood. A marked rise in blood sugar stimulates the pancreas to overproduce insulin, which leads to a hypoglycemic state as too much sugar is transported out of the blood.

Individualize the diet to the patient, since hypoglycemic reactions may occur at any time for various reasons. For example, meal skipping, inadequate calorie intake with excessive energy expenditure, and drinking alcohol may precipitate a low-blood-sugar reaction.

The foods may be divided into three to six or more small meals. Liberal amounts of protein and fat are used, as they are more slowly digested and absorbed. The diet includes meats, fish, poultry, cheese, eggs, fats, low-starch vegetables, and limited amounts of unsweetened fruit and juices, breads, cereals, and high-starch-content vegetables (like corn, peas, and potatoes).

Because milk contains the sugar lactose, limit it to 2 cups a day for an adult. Sweets such as candy, sugar, jams, jellies, soft drinks, and pastries should be avoided to help prevent hypoglycemic reactions. They should be consumed only when necessary to quickly increase blood-sugar levels during a hypoglycemic reaction. If reactions are frequent, it is helpful to carry hard candy for quick and easy use. Handy high-protein snacks to help prevent hypoglycemic reactions may include cheese, peanut butter, milk, and hard-boiled eggs.

Fulfilling the daily requirement of eating a wide variety of foods, in the correct amounts, will contribute directly to a healthy lifestyle. Well-nourished crew members with good health are much more able to resist infections, are able to sleep soundly and awake with a pleasant demeanor. By using your knowledge of diet therapy and nutrition to train and treat your crew, your job will be made significantly easier.

Education and Learning Depend on Good Nutrition and Health

Nutritional and health status are powerful influences on a child's learning and on how well a child performs in school. Children who lack certain nutrients in their diet, or who suffer from protein-energy malnutrition, hunger, parasitic infections or other diseases, do not have the same potential for learning as healthy and well-nourished children. Weak health and poor nutrition among school-age children diminish their cognitive development either through physiological changes or by reducing their ability to participate in learning experiences - or both. Contrary to conventional wisdom, nutritional status does not improve with age.

The extra demands on school-age children (to perform chores, for example, or walk long distances to school) create a need for energy that is much greater than that of younger children. Indeed available data indicate high levels of protein-energy malnutrition and short-term hunger among school-age children. Moreover, deficiencies of critical nutrients such as iodine, vitamin A and iron among the schoolaged are pervasive. It is estimated that 60 million school-age children suffer from iodine deficiency disorders and that another 85 million are at risk for acute respiratory disease and other infections because they are deficient in vitamin A.

The number suffering from iron deficiency anemia is greater still - 210 million. Parasitic worms that infect the intestines or the blood are a major source of disease and malnutrition in school-age children. An estimated 320 million school-age children are infected with roundworm, 233 million with whipworm, and 239 million with hookworm. Schistosomiasis affects an estimated 200 million people throughout the world, approximately 88 million of whom are under 15 years old.

Poor nutrition and health among schoolchildren contributes to the inefficiency of the educational system. Children with diminished cognitive abilities and sensory impairments naturally perform less well and are more likely to repeat grades and to drop out of school than children who are not impaired; they also enroll in school at a later age, if at all, and finish fewer years of schooling.

The irregular school attendance of malnourished and unhealthy children is one of the key factors in poor performance. Even temporary hunger, common in children who are not fed before going to school, can have an adverse effect on learning. Children who are hungry have more difficulty concentrating and performing complex tasks, even if otherwise well nourished. Research and program experience shows that improving nutrition and health can lead to better performance, fewer repeated grades and reduced drop out.

School Feeding Programs: Improve Educational Quality and Efficiency

School Feeding Programs (SFPs) are one of several

interventions that can address some of the nutrition and health problems of school-age children. SFPs, and other school-based nutrition and health programs, can also motivate parents to enroll their children in school and to see that they attend regularly. Experience shows that properly designed and effectively implemented SFPs can:

— *Alleviate short-term hunger in malnourished or otherwise well-nourished schoolchildren.* This helps to increase the attention and concentration of students producing gains in cognitive function and learning.

— *Motivate parents to enroll their children in school and have them attend regularly.* When programs effectively reduce absenteeism and increase the duration of schooling, educational outcomes (performance, dropout, and repetition) improve.

— *Address specific micronutrient deficiencies in school-age children.* Most important of these are iodine and iron, which directly affect cognition. Meeting the iron and iodine needs of school-age children can translate into better school performance.

— *Increase community involvement in schools,* particularly where programs depend on the community to prepare and serve meals to children. Schools with their communities behind them are more effective than schools with less community involvement.

Alleviate Short-term Hunger and Improve Cognition

The number of hungry school-age children is unknown, but is likely to be a significant problem in various circumstances. Many factors contribute to hunger in schoolchildren : the long distances children have to travel to school, cultural meal practices that include no or small breakfasts or a lack of family time or resources to provide adequate meals to children before and/or during the school day. Simply alleviating this hunger in schoolchildren helps them to perform better in school.

— In Jamaica providing breakfast to primary school students significantly increased attendance and arithmetic scores. The children who benefited most were those who were wasted, stunted, or previously malnourished.

— A US study showed the benefits of providing breakfast to disadvantaged primary school students. Before the start of a school breakfast program, eligible (low-income) children scored significantly lower on achievement testes than those not eligible. Once in the program, however, the test scores of the children participating in the program improved more than the scores of non-participants. The attendance of participating children also improved.

— In Peru 23 malnourished and 29 well-nourished 9 to 11 year old boys were studied to assess the effects of breakfast on cognitive performance. Each boy served as his own control in a manner comparable to the Jamaica study cited above. Breakfast was a nutritionally fortified beverage and a baked grain product fortified with iron, similar to the meal provided in the government-sponsored school breakfast program. A series of cognitive tests were administered in an experimental setting. Speed in performing a short-term memory test and discrimination of geometric patterns were improved under the breakfast condition in both groups. The effect was more pronounced in the nutritionally disadvantaged children.

Increase Enrollments and Improve Attendance

Children in poor health start school later in life or not at all. A study in Nepal found that the probability of attending school was 5% for stunted children versus 27% for children of normal nutritional status. In Ghana malnourished children entered school at a later age and completed fewer years of school than better nourished children. The number of days that a child attends school is related to cognition and performance.

SFPs can have a positive effect on rates of enrollment and attendance.

— A recent evaluation of an on-going school feeding program in Burkina Faso found that school canteens were associated with increased school enrollment, regular attendance, consistently lower repeater rates, lower dropout rates in disadvantaged provinces, and higher success rates on national exams, especially among girls.

— A small pilot school feeding program in Malawi was evaluated for its effect on enrollment and attendance. Over a three month period there was a 5% increase in enrollment and up to 36% improvement in attendance/ absenteeism compared to control schools over the same period.

— Niger has one of the five lowest school enrollment rates in the world; the school feeding program is intended to enhance attendance of nomad and transhumant families, particularly of girls. Beneficiaries receive the equivalent of the total daily recommended food intake (2,079kcal) in three meals per day. In addition, as an incentive for girls' participation in schools, some families receive an additional take-home ration. Evidence from past experience with the SFP shows that it contributes to its objectives: whenever canteens have been closed, even provisionally, immediate and high absenteeism follows and children are withdrawn from school. In areas with nomadic and transhumant populations, the school year cannot commence until food stocks arrive.

Although not a school feeding program in the traditional sense, school-based food distribution has also been used successfully to improve enrollment and attendance among school-age children, particularly girls.

— In Bangladesh a program of school-based food distribution increased enrollment by 20% versus a 2% decline in non-participating schools.

— In Pakistan, a program provides an income transfer in the form of one or two tins of oil to families whose girls attend school for 20 days per month. In its pilot phase the oil incentive program demonstrated that it could make a significant contribution to full attendance. In participating schools enrollment improved by 76% compared to 14% in the province overall. Attendance increased from 73% to 95% among participants. The program also claims to put additional food into the hands of mothers and to serve as a contact between mothers and teachers on distribution days.

These food transfer mechanisms do not offer the same potential benefits, for example, meeting short-term hunger and specific nutritional needs, as programs that deliver food directly to beneficiaries. These kinds of programs should therefore be assessed within the context of other food and resource transfer programs.

Micronutrient Deficiencies and Improve Learning

Deficiencies of iron and iodine are among the most harmful types of malnutrition with regard to cognition. Iron deficiency renders children listless, inattentive and uninterested in learning. The research literature suggests a causal link between iron deficiency anemia and less than optimal behavior for learning. Poor performance on a wide range of achievement tests among iron deficient children in school has been consistently documented. Remediation of iron deficiency through supplementation has eliminated the differences in school performance and IQ scores between schoolchildren previously deficient in iron and those without iron deficiencies.

In the case of iodine, most studies have focussed on the differences in cognitive test performance between children who lived in communities with and without endemic goiter. The results show differences in favor of the non-goiter areas. In Sicily, the proportion of children with below-normal cognitive scores was 3% in areas with sufficient iodine, 18.5% in areas where iodine was inadequate, and 19.3% where iodine was inadequate and cretinism was endemic. Studies in Indonesia and Spain have documented similar effects on children in areas with insufficient iodine.

Fortification of school rations is the most efficient and effective route to alleviating micronutrient deficiencies in schoolchildren where SFPs are in operation.

— In South Africa, soup fortified with iron and vitamin C was provided to 350 schools in an area of low socio-economic development on the Cape Peninsula. Results showed that initially 12% of six to seven year old and 20% of 8 to 12 year old children had low weight-for-age, and 49% and 31% had low serum ferritin (a measure of iron deficiency) respectively. At follow-up, after 15 weeks of intervention, iron status improved significantly; falling from 49% to 28% in 6 to 7 year old children and 31% to 21% in 8 to 12 year old children.

— A relatively new breakfast program in Peru, which includes an iron-fortified ration, was evaluated for its short-term impact on diet, amongst other factors. The program significantly increased dietary intakes of energy by 25%, protein by 28% and iron by 46%.

— A case-control study of the impact of providing heme-fortified cookies to school children in Chile found higher concentrations of hemoglobin among children receiving the fortified cookies through the school lunch program. The impact was most significant among children with greater demands for iron such as post-menarchial girls and pubertal boys.

Promote Community Participation

Schools that depend on the community to organize and implement SFPs offer certain advantages. These advantages include: increasing the contact, and hence communication, between parents and teachers, officials and others; giving parents the opportunity to become more aware of what goes on at schools; and serving to raise the value of education/the school for parents and the whole community. For example, school canteens are viewed as an important feature of education policy in Morocco. Since 1978 WFP and the government have supported school feeding. The programs have strong government and community support and are viewed as part of a necessary package of inputs for improving education. The feeding program is credited with helping to maintain high enrollment and attendance and encouraging community participation in education. School cooperatives support the school canteens and parents associations assist with the transportation of food aid.

Seven Steps in Developing School Feeding Programs that Improve Education

The research and program literature on SFPs shows the potential that school feeding has to contribute to improving education. These guidelines provide seven recommendations for improving the design and implementation of programs in order to meet some of this potential. The first recommendation, which calls for the establishment of a policy and objectives for school feeding programming, will provide the framework for implementing the subsequent recommendations. These focus on the most critical aspects of school feeding programming including targeting, cost and financing issues, ration composition and meal delivery, program implementation, and monitoring and evaluation, and on the integration of feeding with other interventions that address the nutrition and health needs of schoolchildren. Specifically, it is recommended that program managers and policy makers:

1. Build a consensus on a policy and objectives that focuses on how school feeding can effectively contribute to improving education and to meeting the nutrition and health needs of school-age children.

Program managers and policy-makers need to agree on what 'problems' or 'situations' the school feeding program will to address, who the program will serve, and which program models are feasible for implementation. School feeding programs are highly visible and as a result often have a significant political dimension, particularly since they can represent a considerable income transfer. This reality should not inhibit establishing a policy and objectives that will take advantage of the substantial potential for improving the impact of SFPs on education.

2. Develop targeting criteria and mechanisms that concentrate program resources on high risk children and communities.

There is a built-in tendency toward universal coverage - providing meals for all schoolchildren - since all children in school throughout the day will require food. Furthermore, program coverage and targeting is always subject to a series of political, logistical, technical and informational constraints. In view of the fact that resources are finite, particularly in the poorest countries, and that providing food is expensive, targeting is a critical element of any effort to improve the impact of a SFP on education. Targeting is essential if the program is to reach families and communities that lack the resources to adequately provide for their school-age children or those that need to be motivated to enroll their children in school and to have them attend more regularly.

3. Analyze and identify alternative financing and cost options for SFPs.

The cost of school feeding programs is a major issue for both governments and donors. Feeding programs of any kind are expensive. Financing may include international assistance, but in all cases available public resources, or the potential to draw on them, are required. Cost alone can indicate little about the value of a SFP but, unfortunately, cost-effectiveness analyses, which assess costs relative to impact on nutrition and education outcomes are for the most part unavailable.

4. Elaborate appropriate guidelines for ration composition and the timing of school meals.

To establish appropriate ration guidelines, program managers and policy makers need to analyze the nutrition and health needs of school-age children. Conditions in the education sector, such as levels of school enrollment, attendance, and performance, the availability of infrastructure and the capacity to implement different kinds of SFPs also need to be assessed. Information is also required on the community's perceptions and capacity to participate in school feeding programs.

5. Identify and address any potential bottlenecks in implementation: such as the availability of supplies and other resources, the appropriateness of cooking practices and the management of private sector inputs.

This recommendation is particularly relevant for a program manager who is already operating a program. Once school feeding programs are in place, altering them can meet strong resistance, however, a range of new experiences is now available that has the potential to alleviate some of the common obstacles to efficient and effective programming. Where a school feeding program already exists, a wealth of information is readily accessible; a critical step towards a better program is to thoroughly analyze this on-going experience.

6. Develop monitoring systems that focus on program processes, that is, how a program is functioning, and institute an evaluation system to assess the impact of the program on specific outcomes.

The need to monitor and evaluate programs is not unique to SFPs, but this recommendation is critical to increasing the impact of SFPs. Despite decades of experience there is a dearth of concrete information on the functioning and effectiveness of school feeding programs. This guide provides a general framework for establishing monitoring and evaluation systems for SFPs.

7. Integrate feeding programs with other interventions that address the primary nutrition and health problems of the school-age population.

Last, but by no means least, the past decade has shown the added value of integrating other nutrition and health interventions with feeding. Specifically recommended are deworming, micronutrient fortification or supplementation, and health nutrition and hygiene education. These interventions are described in more detail in Class Action: Improving School Performance in the Developing World through Better Health and Nutrition and in the publications of the Partnership for Child Development.

Policy and Objectives of SFP

Although many SFPs have been conceived out of ideological, political and economic pressures, the prejudices of international or national personnel, or even commercial or other non-objective influences, the first step toward an effective program is to build programs on sound and transparent objectives. Since SFPs are highly visible and can offer a significant income transfer to families they will always be inherently political. To avoid the use of programs for political purposes, information on programs - especially, who the program is for and why and targeting measures- must be made readily available to the public.

Policy development and setting the objectives of school feeding provides the framework for implementing all the other recommendations aimed at improving the contribution that a SFP can make to education and better health and nutrition. The process of policy development calls for compiling information on: what 'food-related' and education-related problems exist in the schoolage population which could be addressed by school feeding; where, geographically, the problems are located; and which school feeding options are available, or could be developed, for addressing these problems.

Policy Development

Analyzing the nutrition and health situation of school-age children has become a way to engage governments in the problems of this age group. The appropriate method of collecting information will vary by needs, circumstances and resources. Techniques include collecting routine statistics, making special surveys, conducting interviews, and holding focus group discussions with parents, teachers, students and health workers. The idea is to generate a rapid assessment of the situation as opposed to implementing a protracted, expensive and bureaucratically complex study. The goal is to quickly grasp the problems and launch a discussion of the possible solutions within the context of the human and financial resources available in any given country.

The goal of targeting is to identify and reach families and communities that lack the resources to adequately provide for their school-age children. If the SFP is intended to motivate families to enroll children in school and to ensure more regular attendance, the target group is families whose children are not in school or who are frequently absent. Mechanisms and criteria for SFP targeting are similar in many cases to those used for other social programs: economic, geographic, and nutrition status. In additicn, specific education criteria such as overall enrollment, female enrollment, absenteeism, or student performance would also be included under some circumstances. In general it appears that SFP targeting is best done at the level of the school, or based on some other criteria - e.g., location - rather than on individual selection. The coverage of SFPs will depend on how many resources are available for programs and on the size of the problem that the program is intended to address.

Targeting Mechanisms

Economic Targeting: Economic or household income targeting is the most difficult of the targeting mechanisms available to implement, since measuring income is not straightforward, particularly where in-kind contributions to family income are substantial. Targeting is dependent on the availability of literate and numerate workers if bureaucratically administered income criteria are to be used.

Community leaders, teachers, local government entities or voluntary organizations can participate in identifying the poorest households, but this requires clear criteria that are transparent and not based on political favoritism. If economic targeting is already in place for other programs, the school program could build on it, however, singling out individual children in a classroom or school for a feeding program or for a reduced price can be stigmatizing and socially and politically unacceptable.

Geographic Targeting: Targeting by geographic area is most commonly used in school feeding programming. By using a poverty map, programming is restricted to certain administrative areas in which people have a high probability of being poor. This type of targeting does not require administrative intervention, but people who are outside of the area may move or travel distances to participate in the program or may enroll their children in those schools. Changing established targeting criteria, usually restricting programs to certain areas, can be difficult and may not be acceptable.

Targeting by Nutrition Status: Targeting SFPs according to nutrition status is usually linked to geographic targeting. A census that records the height and age of first grade children can quickly and easily identifying geographic areas at risk for malnutrition. It obtains these results at low cost - about 10 US cents per child - and can be implemented within a few months. Census results can also be used to target other social programs, in addition to school programs, increasing the benefits of the census relative to its cost. The census can also provide an updated register of schools, including the number of first grade children and their age at entry. This census technique may be less valuable for targeting programs in countries where malnutrition is widespread. It is not recommended to use the height census to select individuals nor is it recommended to do nutrition screening in schools exclusively for a school feeding program. The height census has been used extensively in Latin America, for example in Guatemala, Honduras and the Dominican Republic, to help pinpoint those regions and areas most in need of SFPs.

Gender Targeting: School feeding programming, particularly that supported by the WFP, has recently concentrated on addressing the need to encourage female enrollment and continuation in both primary and secondary school. Toward this end programs are not only targeted at specific regions within countries where female participation in school is a problem, but the ration provided to girls may be of higher nutritional and caloric content to serve as an even greater incentive for girls to attend and stay in school. In some cases the continuation of WFP-assisted programs is contingent on a certain proportion of girls participating in the program.

Analyze the Cost and Financing

SFPs, by virtue of the fact that they include food, are expensive. Beyond the costs of the food itself, the costs associated with food management, logistics and control can represent a significant financial burden for governments. On-site feeding is costly as it requires daily preparation and delivery of food, but is also a model that can invite, or require, community participation. In response to the difficulties of on-site feeding and a new focus on delivering an appropriately-timed (with regard to effecting improvements in learning capacity) and high quality, consistent ration, some countries are developing program models that include less costly commodities and more efficient systems for delivery to schools. Programs that make good use of the education infrastructure for delivery and logistics will be most efficient.

The very fact that SFPs do not require, for the most part, additional infrastructure means that they can be less costly than other types of feeding programs which distribute benefits to groups that are not in one location. Programs that finance expensive kitchen equipment and supplies or build new infrastructure/canteens, however, will significantly raise the costs and lower the relative cost-effectiveness of programs.

Finding ways to minimize implementation problems, particularly food losses, either to spoilage, to the black market or leakage, will help to ensure the financial feasibility of programs. Some SFPs are intentionally designed as an income-transfer for families, especially those that are trying to help attract girls to schools; the benefit received by families from these programs must therefore surpass the costs of having their daughters away from home attending school.

What do Programmes Cost

A comparison of the costs of SFPs is problematic; the number of feeding days varies, as does the quantity of the rations and their quality. In the early 1990s two sizable studies made some accurate comparisons of cross-country cost information by standardizing and controlling for some of these differences. In one instance the data show that the cost of SFPs ranges from US$19.25 to US$208.59 per 1,000 calories per student per day for 365 days. The mean program cost was US$88.74, the median US$81.46. These costs were found to be comparable to those of other types of feeding programs.

A study of feeding programs in Latin America provides the other major source of summary data of standardized school feeding costs. In this analysis of 16 SFPs, delivering 1,000 kcal, cost between US$0.03 and US$0.84; most were around US$0.30. The cost for 100 grams of protein, another way to value the food delivered, ranged from US$0.04 to US$2.07, with milk at the extreme high end of the scale.

An analysis of three donor-assisted SFPs in Burkina Faso, Cape Verde and the Gambia show the range of costs associated with these SFPs. Consistent with the Horton research, the three programs cost between US$43.12 and US$171.43 per 1,C00 kcal per student per day for 365 days/year. This analysis included the cost of the programs without the value of the food since the food does not represent an actual outlay for the countries. This calculation yields standardized program costs ranging from US$17.24 to US$56.05 per pupil per year. Unlike these donor-assisted programs, some governments are developing and supporting SFP models that draw on the lessons learned regarding the timing of meals, alternative delivery mechanisms, decentralized management and the integration of other interventions with feeding. These programs are only in the early stages so that actual program data is unavailable, but for comparison it is useful to look at the proposed/ budgeted food costs for these new programs.

Financing and Cost Issues

Food Aid: Food aid is an important source of support for SFPs. There are high costs associated with transportation, warehouses and distribution; adequate storage facilities are required at every stage from port to the point of distribution. These costs are often borne by recipient governments. Management and distribution of food requires trained people to keep track of food inventories and their location, human resources may be as much of a constraint as cash and physical facilities. Nonetheless, if the economic and financial costs are acceptable then the cost of these programs may not be prohibitive relative to the benefit provided.

Private Sector: Drawing on the private sector for school feeding programming overcomes many of the difficulties of on-site preparation of meals, and may be one of the least costly ways to feed children in schools. The private sector in this case can be street vendors, local canteen or a large canteen company. However, even these programs incur costs in monitoring and supervision, and the start-up costs for developing school meal alternatives and making arrangements with vendors can be substantial. Programs that utilize school canteens or street food vendors for school-based feeding programs may offer the most economical approach to school feeding. However, the technical and logistical implications, and hence costs in training and supplies to improve the provision of food through these sources are not insubstantial. Remarkably little concrete analysis has been done on this approach to school feeding.

Food Selections: Certain food selections are particularly expensive; foremost among these is milk, which is expensive per the number of calories, and nutrients it provides, and is perishable, which if figured in with the cost increases costs even further. UHT milk alternatives, which overcome the perishability issues, are particularly expensive to produce, especially in developing countries where the relevant technology is not widespread.

Community Support: Parent-teacher or other community associations can play a significant role in a SFP and ultimately assume some of the costs. Efforts to strengthen parent-teacher organizations and increase the links between communities and schools are highly recommended.

Targeting: Where feasible, more refined targeting mechanisms that maximize the participation of the most needy populations improve the efficiency of programs. Ultimately this can mean charging fees to students who can afford them for participation in the program.

Sustainability: Food transfer programs cannot be considered 'sustainable' in the same way as, for example, a revolving credit program, which ultimately pays for itself. A continual input of resources is required in order to provide food for school children. From the donor point of view, a program may be seen as sustainable if the government commits to continuing the program after donor support is removed. From the perspective of the individual beneficiary, the sustainable aspect of the program is likely to be the lasting impact on behavior changes brought about through education or other interventions that are part of the program.

Determine Optimal Rations and Timing of Meals

The 'best ration' and when to deliver it depends on the program's objective. School meals provided early in the school day to alleviate hunger before or while classes are in session should help to improve attention, concentration, and achievement among children. Historically, and even now, political and social objectives dominate in school feeding programming. School meals were viewed, and in many cases still are, as a means for a school child to receive a large meal in the middle of the day, which typically coincides with local dietary practices.

These programs served, and continue to serve, not only as nutrition programs, but perhaps more as social welfare programs that provide a substantial economic benefit to the family since the child will not eat at mid-day from the family pot. Nonetheless, the nutritional quality and quantity of a ration should always be assessed as well as the effects of the timing of ration delivery. Other factors such as local food habits, logistical considerations, food availability, and cost will also influence the selection of the ratior.. General ration guidelines that can be applied almost universally are:

— A school snack or meal usually provides from one-third to one-half of the recommended daily allowance for energy and protein for the school-age group targeted by the program. A substantial ration is recommended to ensure overcompensating in order that parents don't withdraw more food at home than the child receives at school. Programs which include older children, particularly adolescents, in the target group will require larger rations to meet the increased nutritional needs during this period (see Table 3).

— Rations that fill the actual micronutrient gaps in the diets of school-age children are higher in nutritional quality and can be expected to have greater impacts on learning (see Table 4). Ensuring that the appropriate level of micronutrients is included in the school ration may require more than selecting the appropriate mix of foods. Fortification may be an option if the size of the ration is relatively small, where the ration itself, or a component like flour, is centrally processed, or where the foods to be used do not contain a high level of the most critical micronutrients.

Table 3: Mean Daily Per Capita Energy Requirement and Safe Protein Intake

	Pre-Primary 3-5 yrs	*Primary 6-12*	*Adolescent 11-14*
Energy (Kcal)	1700	1900	2350
Protein (grams)	32	40	46

Table 4: Recommended Mean Daily Intakes for Vitamin A, Iron and Iodine

Age group	*Vitamin A retinol/IU)*	*(ug Iron (mg)*	*Iodine (ug)*
Pre-primary (1-6)	400/1330	10	90
Primary (7-10)	400/1330	10	120
Adolescents	500/1665	12	
	(10-12yrs)	(boys 11-14yrs)	150
	600/2000	15	
	(12-15yrs)	(girls 11-14yrs)	

— Fresh milk, although it appears to be nutritious and convenient, is not recommended as it is usually an expensive source of calories and is perishable and subject to contamination.

— A meal or snack provided early in the school day will eliminate hunger so that children are more attentive in class.

Simplify Program Implementation

On-site prepared meals, pre-prepared meals and food in bulk or coupons are the primary school feeding program models. Each model is associated with a different set of issues related to program implementation.

In many cases the current emphasis on the timing of meals - providing the school meal early in the day to maximize the impact of the program on educational objectives- involves a significant change from current practice. Furthermore, given the conditions for meal preparation in many developing countries - e.g., the need to utilize volunteers, long distances to fetch water and fuel for cooking, slow cooking facilities - the successful preparation and provision of meals to children early in the day is not easy. New program approaches have recently been developed and tested to overcome some of the technical and logistical obstacles associated with SFPs that countries might consider in developing new and modifying on-going programs:

— *Use of snack foods:* Providing a snack as opposed to what may be a more traditional school meal (school lunch) will significantly cut the preparation time. In Indonesia, for example, a new program will provide from 10 to 15 US cents per ration for the local production of a snack food with 300 kcal and 5 grams of protein. The intent of this program is specifically to avoid industrially produced snack foods, since another objective is to increase local food production, however, the emphasis is equally on the delivery of an appropriately-timed snack. The basic foods to be used are tubers (cassava sweet potato, taro), cereals (rice, corn), fruits, and vegetables. Snack foods also avoid the problem of substitution of the school meal for one of the family meals; this is preferable from a nutritional perspective since the school meal will be additional to the normal diet.

— *Products with quicker cooking times:* Blended foods and cereal flours can be prepared much more quickly than unmilled whole grains. In Kenya, for example, a long-running program that provided a school lunch to children involved more than 4 hours of preparation time. A recent pilot program which substituted the traditional meal of maize, beans, bread, vegetable oil etc. for a program which provided an early morning drink and biscuits and a midday porridge, made with a blended food, effectively cut the preparation time to less than an hour. Unfortunately, although the foods were readily accepted and there were savings in fuel costs, this saving was canceled out by the 35% higher cost for transportation since the shelf life of products was much shorter.

— *Monetization:* Monetization is the sale of donated foods in the general market so that the central government can give the proceeds to school systems for feeding programs; the school systems then purchase the food in their local communities. This practice obviates the need to transport large quantities of food around countries, which in many cases is a severe obstacle to implementing consistent and effective programs. It also can increase the choice of food commodities that can be used in the feeding program. This practice is becoming increasingly popular. Although it generates income for the local economy, putting donated food in the market can depress indigenous food production and increase the risk of mismanagement and corruption. Issues of food preparation also need to be addressed.

— *The private sector:* The off-site prepared meal/snack program addresses many of the technical and logistical concerns of SFPs. Programs in Peru and the Dominican Republic are examples of the private sector approach to school meals. In both cases the meal provided is a snack or breakfast which is itself a break from the traditional school lunch. Utilizing private enterprises to prepare and deliver the snack foods to schools facilitates the provision of the ration early in the day as well as ensuring a consistent and high quality ration while taking a minimal time away from learning. One problem with these programs can be the monotony of the ration.

— *The informal private sector/street vendors:* Enlisting the support of local street vendors to provide better quality school meals to children is an option to consider. In Lesotho, for example, former local vendors who successfully bid to provide the privatized service run school canteens. In Nigeria, state and local governments train and license vendors who sell to schoolchildren. In other cases school principals exercise their authority locally and choose the vendors to serve their schools. A major concern that must be addressed in using this option is the quality and hygiene of the food served.

— *Information, education and communication (IEC) campaigns:* Effective IEC programs which promote understanding of the benefits of providing meals earlier in the day and encourage the practices needed to realize early meal preparation, while addressing resistance to this approach, will help to encourage change to more cost-effective programs. Furthermore, it may be possible to alleviate hunger in schoolchildren without a formal feeding program. Encouraging and educating parents to feed their children before sending them to school or to provide a bag lunch or money for them to purchase food while at school may be an appropriate objective for IEC campaigns.

Ensure Useful Monitoring of Processes and Evaluation of Outcomes

Programme Monitoring

The purpose of program monitoring is to refine and optimize the approach to delivering the SFP to the beneficiaries. The monitoring system is not intended to assess the impact of a program, but to assess how consistently a program is operated relative to its design. The intention is to gather information that will help program administrators and participants to assess program operation. Such monitoring would ideally lead to the identification of bottlenecks in program operation and to suggestions of areas for improvement. It would inform program implementers, in particular, on the 'nuts and bolts' of program operation, such as:

— how many children are reached and where;

— what level of inputs are being delivered: number of meals served, calories delivered, micronutrients received;

— the quality and quantity of the activities under the SFP, for example, the training or education programs for staff and teachers, food storage and inventory practices, the organization and participation of the community in the program;

— how much is being spent in the various elements of the program.

Evaluation

The evaluation of a SFP entails looking at the impact of the program on some aspect of children's lives, for example, nutrition status, learning or school performance. The purpose of evaluating an on-going program is to explore what the effects of the program have been, to review how things have changed since the program has been in operation and to determine if the program has made a difference. Program evaluation is intended to contribute to informed decisions that could lead to the continuation of the program in its current form, discontinuation of the program or to changes/ improvements in the design. The indicators or measures of program performance to use in program evaluation will vary in each particular situation; availability of data will vary as will the capacity of local personnel and institutions. The expected impact of a particular program - the purpose of a SFP - will also vary; for example, those that are aimed at improving gender issues versus those that emphasize alleviation of short-term hunger in all children. Nevertheless, experience suggests that the following general guidelines can be usefully applied in the evaluation of SFPs:

— Indicators that are simple and feasible (in terms of ease of collection) are best. If local implementers cannot easily collect and analyze evaluation data then the system will not be useful.

— Where reliable and valid achievement and learning measures are not built into schools, proxy indicators for student learning can be devised. Attendance data is a proxy for learning; the research is clear that children who attend school more regularly learn more. Since attendance data is usually only available at the level of the school it is difficult to obtain. It is important to check the validity and reliability of this data and it would be useful to explore the possibility of collecting additional proxies for learning, such as classroom observations in a sample of schools, to assist in validating the attendance data.

— Gender-specific enrollment and other school data such as pupil flow (dropout, repetition) which is usually centrally collated may be easier to access. This data represents important measures for assessing program impact particularly where programs are intended to address gender issues. However, there tends to be a risk of substantial subjectivity in the measurement of these outcomes.

— Simple tools to assess health status in children - e.g. height-for-age, prevalence of parasitic infection - can also be used to demonstrate the impact of programs.

Seek Opportunities for Integrated Interventions

Offering other school-based health and nutrition interventions in addition to food can boost the educational and nutritional value of SFPs. Treating children for parasites, for example, can improve both their appetites and the nutritional benefit of the food ration. If the ration is not a good source of nutrients or adequately fortified with them, the SFP can be used to deliver micronutrient supplements. Nutrition and health education aimed at changing specific nutrition and health practices could also enhance the benefits of SFPs.

Key Interventions

School-based helminth control: School-based helminth control delivers deworming drugs to children through schools in areas where infection is common without screening individuals for infection. Treatment is inexpensive, safe, easy to deliver, and highly cost-effective. Bypassing the need for screening not only decreases cost but also increases compliance because some children choose to avoid the diagnostic procedure, which requires collection of a stool sample. Moreover because school-age children typically harbor the most intense helminth infections, treatment of this group is one of the best ways to reduce infection in the entire community. Integrating helminth control with SFPs is becoming a popular way to address this significant health problem of schoolage children as well as to increase the value of the school meal.

Micronutrient supplementation: As with school-based helminth control programs, school-based micronutrient supplementation programs are based on the premise that a large proportion of children are deficient in certain micronutrients, especially iron, iodine and vitamin A, and supplements can be easily and inexpensively delivered in a school setting. The costs of the micronutrients are quite low and if integrated with the delivery system of a SFP, no additional delivery costs need be incurred. Fortification of school rations remains the best alternative to alleviating micronutrient deficiencies where this is possible. If deficiency problems are particularly severe or other factors inhibit the fortification of the ration, supplementation is the next best choice until fortification through the regular food supply is possible and widespread.

Information, education, communication (IEC): Inappropriate behavior by school-age children, such as playing in or drinking impure water, is the basis of many nutrition and health problems. Education that addresses specific nutrition and health practices is a critical element of school nutrition and health programs, including SFPs. Such education complements, and can help sustain, the benefits of short-to medium-term interventions such as deworming and micronutrient supplementation, which will in turn increase the benefits of SFPs. In addition, as mentioned earlier, IEC programs are important for promoting needed changes in SFPs and addressing resistances to these changes.

4

Malnutrition and Adulteration

Nutrition is defined as the science or study of the appropriate diet to promote health. Nutrition also refers to the intake of food and other essentials for promoting growth and replacing or repairing worn or damaged tissue. Nutrition plays a vital part in our wellness, health promotion, disease prevention and rehabilitation. Nutrients support metabolism of all cells thereby sustaining life as we know it. Proper cellular functioning depends on at least 50 essential nutritional compounds and elements. Disease and death may occur if only one of these essential nutrients is deficient or excessive. Nutritional screening is a good first step to take when addressing the nutrition-related problems amount older adults.

Malnutrition refers to an inappropriate or improper intake of food and other essentials The World Health Organization defines malnutrition as "the cellular imbalance between supply of nutrients and energy and the body's demand for them to ensure growth, maintenance, and specific functions." Protein-energy malnutrition (PEM), first described in the 1920s, is observed most frequently in developing countries.

Causes of Malnutrition

Factors that contribute to high rates of malnutrition include:

— Bad eating habits

— Dental problems

— Lack of nutrition knowledge

— Depression

— Social isolation

— Poverty

— Sensory losses

— Age-related changes

Poor nutrition can lead to a number of health-related problems. They include:

— Cognitive dysfunction

— Depressed immune function (which leads to an increased risk of infection and slower wound healing)

— Anemia

— Fatigue

— Orthostatic hypotension (a drop in blood pressure when standing up that can lead to fainting)

— Increased risk of hip fracture

— Decreased muscle strength

— Pressure sores

— Swelling of the feet and ankles

— Depressed thyroid function

— Increased risk of detrimental drug interactions

Inadequate food intake is the most common cause of malnutrition worldwide. In developing countries, inadequate food intake is secondary to insufficient or inappropriate food supplies. Inadequate sanitation further endangers children by increasing the risk of infectious diseases that increase nutritional losses and metabolic demands.

In developed countries, inadequate food intake is a less common cause of malnutrition. Instead, diseases and, in particular, chronic illnesses play an important role in the etiology of malnutrition. Children with chronic illness are at risk for nutritional problems for several reasons, including the following:

— Children with chronic illnesses frequently have anorexia, which leads to inadequate food intake.

— Increased inflammatory burden and increased metabolic demands can increase caloric need.

— Any chronic illness that involves the liver or small bowel affects nutrition adversely by impairing digestive and absorptive functions.

Chronic illnesses that commonly are associated with nutritional deficiencies include the following:

— Cystic fibrosis

— Chronic renal failure

— Childhood malignancies

— Congenital heart disease

— Neuromuscular diseases

Chilaren with multiple food allergies present a special nutritional challenge because of severe dietary restrictions. Patients with active allergic symptoms may have increased calorie and protein needs.

Signs and Symptoms of Under- and Over-nutrition

Clinical signs and symptoms of PEM include the following:

— Poor weight gain

— Slowing of linear growth

— Behavioral changes - Irritability, apathy, decreased social responsiveness, anxiety, and attention deficits

Some of the clinical signs and symptoms of specific micronutrient deficiencies may closely resemble those observed in PEM. Deficiencies of micronutrients, including vitamins, minerals, and trace elements have been well described. The most common and clinically significant deficiencies include the following:

Iron	Fatigue, anemia, decreased cognitive function, headache, glossitis, and nail changes
Iodine	Goiter, developmental delay, and mental retardation
Vitamin D	Poor growth, rickets, and hypocalcemia
Vitamin A	Night blindness, xerophthalmia, poor growth, and hair changes
Folate	Glossitis, anemia (megaloblastic), and neural tube defects (in fetuses of women without folate supplementation)

Physical: Physical findings that are associated with PEM include the following:

— *Decreased subcutaneous tissue*: Areas that are most affected are the legs, arms, buttocks, and face.

— *Edema*: Areas that are most affected are the distal extremities and anasarca [generalized edema].

— Oral changes

— Cheilosis

— Angular stomatitis

— Papillar atrophy

— Abdominal findings

— Abdominal distension secondary to poor abdominal musculature

— Hepatomegaly secondary to fatty infiltration

— Skin changes

— Dry peeling skin with raw exposed areas
— Hyperpigmented plaques over areas of trauma
— *Nail changes*: Nails become fissured or ridged.
— *Hair changes*: Hair is thin, sparse, brittle, easily pulled out, and turns a dull brown or reddish color.

Pathophysiology

Malnutrition affects virtually every organ system. Dietary protein is needed to provide amino acids for synthesis of body proteins and other compounds that have a variety of functional roles. Energy is essential for all biochemical and physiologic functions in the body. Furthermore, micronutrients are essential in many metabolic functions in the body as components and cofactors in enzymatic processes.

In addition to the impairment of physical growth and of cognitive and other physiologic functions, immune response changes occur early in the course of significant malnutrition in a child. These immune response changes correlate with poor outcomes and mimic the changes observed in children with acquired immune deficiency syndrome (AIDS). Loss of delayed hypersensitivity, fewer T lymphocytes, impaired lymphocyte response, impaired phagocytosis secondary to decreased complement and certain cytokines, and decreased secretory immunoglobulin A (IgA) are some changes that may occur.

Frequency

The World Health Organization estimates that approximately 150 million children (26.7%) younger than 5 years in developing countries are malnourished based on their low weight in relation to their age. An additional 200 million children have stunted height secondary to poor nutrition. More than half of young children in South Asia have PEM, which is 5 times the prevalence in the Western Hemisphere. In sub-

Saharan Africa, 30% of children have PEM. Two thirds of all malnourished children in the world live in Asia, and another one fourth live in Africa.

Mortality/Morbidity

The adverse effects of malnutrition include physical and developmental manifestations. Poor weight gain and slowing of linear growth occur. Impairment of immunologic functions in these children mimics those observed in children with AIDS, predisposing them to opportunistic and other typical childhood infections.

Children who are chronically malnourished exhibit behavioral changes, including irritability, apathy and decreased social responsiveness, anxiety, and attention deficits. In addition, infants and young children who have malnutrition frequently demonstrate developmental delay or permanent cognitive deficits. The degree of delay and deficit depends on the severity and duration of nutritional compromise and the age at which malnutrition occurs. In developing countries, approximately 50% of the 10 million deaths each year are secondary to malnutrition in children younger than 5 years.

Age

Children are most vulnerable to the effects of malnutrition in infancy and early childhood. Premature infants have special nutritional needs that are not met with traditional feeding recommendations; they require fortified human milk or specially designed preterm formula until later in infancy. Children are susceptible to malnutrition for differing reasons. During adolescence, self-imposed dietary restrictions contribute to the incidence of nutritional deficiencies.

Adverse Effects of Malnutrition

Kwashiorkor and marasmus are 2 forms of PEM that are wide spreaded. The distinction between the 2 forms of PEM is based on the presence (kwashiorkor) or absence (marasmus) of edema. Marasmus involves inadequate intake of protein and calories, whereas a child with kwashiorkor has fair-to-normal calorie intake with inadequate protein intake. Although significant clinical differences between kwashiorkor and marasmus exist, some studies suggest that marasmus represents an adaptation to starvation whereas kwashiorkor represents a dysadaptation to starvation.

In addition to PEM, children may be affected by micronutrient deficiencies, which also have a detrimental effect on growth and development. The most common and clinically significant micronutrient deficiencies in children and childbearing women throughout the world include deficiencies of iron, iodine, folate, vitamin D, and vitamin A.

Although fortification programs have helped diminish deficiencies of iodine, vitamin A, and vitamin D in individuals in the United States, these deficiencies remain a significant cause of morbidity in developing countries. Micronutrient deficiencies and protein and calorie deficiencies must be addressed for optimal growth and development to be attained in these individuals.

The nutrient deficiency caused by malnutrition and the related physical manisfestation are listed in table 1.

Table 1. Nutrient deficiency and physical manisfestation

Nutrient Deficiency	Physical Manisfestation
Protein	Edema, hypoalbuminemia; enlarged liver; diarrhea
Protein/Energy	Muscle wasting; sparse, thin dry, brittle hair; dry, inelastic skin; muscle weakness
Vitamin A	Poor visual accommodation to dark; Bitot's spots (eyes); dryness of the eyes; hair loss; impaired taste; gooseflesh
Vitamin D	Bowed legs, beading of ribs, and other skeletal deformities (Rickets)

Vitamin K	Bleeding (poor coagulation of blood)
Thiamin (B1)	Cardiac enlargement, mental confusion; irritability; calf muscle tenderness and foot drop; hypoflexia; hyperesthesia; parethesia
Riboflavin (B2)	Fissures around mouth; reddened, scaly, greasy skin around the nose and mouth; magenta-colored tongue
Niacin (B3)	Bright red, swollen, painful tongue; Pellagrous dermatitis; Depression, insomnia, headaches, dizziness; dementia; diarrhea
Pyriodoxine (B6)	Neuropathies; Glossitis; Nasolabial seborrhea
Folic Acid	Red, painful, shiny, smooth tongue; skin hyperpigmentation
Vitamin B12	Mild dementia; sensory losses in hands and feet; red, smooth, shiny, painful tongue; mild jaundice; optic neuritis; anorexia; diarrhea
Vitamin C	Joint tenderness and swelling; hemorrhages under the skin; spongy gums that bleed easily; poor wound healing; petechiae
Fatty Acids	Sparse hair growth; dry flaky skin; depression and psychosis; dementia
Calcium	Poor reflexes; poor cardiovascular accommodation to activity; slow mental processing; depression; dementia
Magnesium	Lethargy and weakness; anorexia and vomiting; tremor; convulsions
Iodine	Goiter
Iron	Pallor; pale, atrophic tongue; spoon-shaped nails; pale conjunctivae
Zinc	Sluggish muscle contraction; poor wound healing; diminshed taste and appetite; dermatitis; hair loss; diarrhea

Deleterious Effects

The two other classical nutrition-related diseases, that is iodine deficiency and fluorosis, give good examples of how well-intentioned developmental programmes could aggravate and deleteriously alter the course of a disease.

Iodine Deficiency Disorders

Iodine deficiency disorders in India had been traditionally considered to be a disease state predominantly confined to the sub-Himalayan hilly regions of the country. Huge pendulous goitres and frank cretinism have been reported from the vast sub-Himalayan belt of the country. Goitre has also been reported from the hilly areas of South-East Asian countries such as Thailand, Myanmar and Indonesia. With the institution of the programme of iodization of common salt, the disease had shown signs of substantial regression in these countries since the 1970s.

Since the 1980s, however, a change in the epidemiology of the disease has become noticeable not only in India but in other South Asian countries as well. The iodine deficiency problem in India seems to have now invaded the irrigated plains and is no longer confined to the hilly regions of the sub-Himalayan tract alone. The goitre that is now widely seen in the irrigated plains is certainly not of the huge pendulous variety but often manifests as a low-grade enlargement of the thyroid gland. Using radioimmunoassay techniques, Kochupillai provides evidence of widespread neonatal hypothyroidism in several thousands of new borns in the plains of India.

The important question for our present purpose is: what are the factors that have led to the changing epidemiology of goitre and its emergence in new areas hitherto not known to be goitre endemic.

The possibilities that need to be considered in the context of the emerging evidence are:

— Intensive irrigation involved as part of the agricultural technology following the Green Revolution has resulted in soil alkalinity and depletion of soil micronutrients. Efforts at correcting this through periodic soil testing and soil repletion have been tardy. Depletion of soil iodine is part of this problem and is reflected in the diminished content of iodine in foods and water. Thus, data from

NIN, Hyderabad have shown that the average iodine content of water from goitrous areas is 3–16 m g/l as against 5–64 m g/l in non-goitrous areas. Iodine content in foods could be as low as 173–265 m g/day. The extensive loss of iodine from the soil is also attributable to intensive multiple cropping. The intensive cultivation of such crops as sugarcane and the resulting loss of iodine from the soil caused by the considerable biomass generated are factors contributing to this loss.

— Fertilizers, pesticides and food additives now widely used could be expected to inhibit iodine utilization.

— Increased urinary thiocynate levels in endemic areas, in the fact of seemingly adequate levels of urinary iodine excretion have raised the possibility of excessive ingestion of goitrogens which may be expected to interfere with the utilization of iodine by the thyroid gland. Such goitrogens could either be of dietary origin or could be in the nature of food contaminants in the environment. Goitrogens have been reported from a wide range of plant foods. The question that has to be decided is whether the concentrations of goitrogens in plant foods, which have been known for a long time, have increased in recent years following the institution of modern intensive agricultural technology? Have the heavy use of fertilizers and the new farming procedures now in vogue contributed to the increased uptake and generation of goitrogens in plant foods? Increased urinary thiocynate levels in some endemic areas point to this possibility.

Fluorosis

Fluorosis was first described in India by Shortt *et al.* more than 60 years ago. The disease had been recognized as an endemic problem in parts of the Punjab, Andhra Pradesh, Karnataka, Rajasthan and Uttar Pradesh. The primary cause of endemic fluorosis had been established to be excessive intake of the element fluoride. Since food items do not contribute much fluoride, it is the amount of fluoride ingested through drinking water that determines the risk of fluorosis. However, it is known that other factors in the food influence the susceptibility to fluorosis. Thus, fluorosis is more common among millet (jowar) eaters than among rice eaters, and the presence of vitamin C and calcium in the diet also appears to be an important determinant.

In children, fluoride toxicity primarily affects the teeth (dental fluorosis). In adults, the bony skeleton, ligaments and tendons are affected. The central pathological process is excessive formation of bone and inappropriate calcification of soft tissues. The subjects afflicted with the disease often suffer from spinal deformities and poker backs and are quite often disabled.

While these clinical manifestations were well recognized, a new and serious dimension to the problems of skeletal fluorosis suddenly emerged in the mid-1970s. NIN, Hyderabad, then discovered that in parts of Andhra Pradesh, which were long known to be endemic for fluorosis, a large number of adolescents and young adults had developed marked degrees of *genu valgum* or 'knock knees' of a form so severe that it incapacitated them. This was an entirely new development seen for the first time in areas where formerly only the classical form of skeletal fluorosis was seen in older men.

In 28 villages belonging to the endemic areas that were surveyed by the NIN team, as many as 600 (2.8 per cent) out of 21,000 subjects surveyed, had this striking deformity. There was also a wide variation between villages with prevalence ranging from as low as 0.2 per cent to 17 per cent. In some villages, almost all the youth were affected.

A series of interesting studies revealed that this new aggravation of an old disease was related to the construction of the large Nagarjunasagar Dam which impounds large amounts of water. The dam had been hailed as a major developmental project which had extended irrigation facilities to a vast, dry and arid area. As part of the developmental effort and in order to mobilize and harness water resources for the increasing population, large dams are being constructed in several developing countries. There is now evidence that in some cases, these well-intentioned efforts could have deleterious consequences. The impounding of water by huge dams could bring about changes in subsoil water levels and in soil chemistry. The sequence of events leading to the new manifestations are stated briefly:

Following the construction of the dam and the impounding of large quantities of water, there was an elevation of levels of subsoil water in the dam vicinity and the rise of soil alkalinity which influences the concentration of trace elements in food grains grown in that area. The concentration of molybdenum in food increases and, in view of the well-known antagonistic relationship between molybdenum and copper, leads to copper deficiency and facilitates bone deformities.

Most importantly, fluoride content in subsoil water and in foods grown in the area had also increased. Thus, *genu valgum* afflicting young adults emerged as a new phenomenon, consequent to the construction of the Nagarjunasagar Dam.

Here then, is an instance of an unforseen ecological repercussion of a well-intentioned development programme which was envisaged as an unmixed blessing that would help irrigate vast tracts of land and help grow more food. This experience in Nagarjunasagar has again been repeated in another part of the country, though not because of the construction of a dam but because of another development programme.

The growing population pressure and the resultant scarcity of drinking water in the country has now led to the policy of providing tube-wells, so that a water source is available within a distance of 200 m of any household (100 m in hilly areas). Millions of tube-wells have been thus provided during the last few decades. Tube-wells were also preferred because of the widespread contamination of surface water with water-borne micro-organisms responsible for cholera and hepatitis. Tube-wells have no doubt contributed to the elimination of water-borne diseases in quite a few areas. However, in some areas where the aquifer is surrounded by fluoride-contaminating earth – cryolite, calcite, fluorospar and mica – the water from the tube-well is contaminated with excess fluoride. Thus, all tube-wells are not safe from the point of view of fluorosis in situations where tube-well water is rich in fluoride, it has become necessary to resort to surface-water sources, after proper treatment of such sources. In areas where excess fluoride has not been detected, an aggravation of fluorosis has been observed.

An epidemiological survey carried out in village Tilaipani, in district Mandla of Mandhya Pradesh, has revealed a high prevalence of *genu valgum* (51.1 per cent) and dental fluorosis (74.4 per cent) among youth below 20 years, while 16.3 per cent of the children below 10 years were also affected with fluorosis. This is again a relatively new development. While in the Nagarjunasagar area of Andhra Pradesh, the construction of a large dam started the chain of events leading to the aggravation of fluorosis, at Mandla in Madhya Pradesh, fluorosis had become aggravated due to the digging of deep bore-wells (more than 42 m deep), and large-scale consumption of water from such deep bore-wells as against surface wells which were in vogue earlier. The first cases of lower limb deformities were observed two years after the first tube-wells were dug. Thereafter, within a span of three years, the number of cases increased in quick succession to reach the present magnitude of 51.1 per cent for *genu valgum*, and 74.4 per cent for dental fluorosis among youth below the age of 20 years. Incidentally, deep tube-wells have also been found to be responsible for the outbreak of arsenicosis in the Malda district of West Bengal.

Overweight and Obesity

By some estimates, 97 million adults or about 55% of Americans are overweight or obese. Being overweight increases the risk for many common chronic diseases, including heart disease, certain cancers, stroke, non-insulin dependent diabetes, and atherosclerosis. Those who are obese have a lower life expectancy and many more health problems. However, for those who are older and overweight, several studies indicate that the relationship between obesity and mortality risk decreases with age.

In earlier decades, gaining weight during middle age was considered acceptable. We know now that even a modest midlife weight gain will significantly increase your risk of heart disease. A study from Harvard that followed nearly 116,000 registered nurses for 14 years found that even weight gain within the "normal" range, as well as modest weight gains after 18 years of age, appears to increase the risk of coronary heart disease in middle-aged women when compared to those who had not gained weight.

The coronary risk rose 25 percent among those who gained 11 to 18 pounds; 60 percent for a weight gain of 18 to 25 pounds and 200 to 300 percent increase for weight gains above 25 pounds. The source of calories—whether a low-fat or more balanced low-calorie diet—did not have much effect on weight, suggesting that it is overeating that is the problem.

Furthermore, this study found that people who exercised regularly are usually able to maintain their weight, which suggests that exercise, not diet, should be the primary focus of efforts. Most experts agree that a combination of reducing calorie intake and increasing physical activity are necessary for weight loss.

Body shape matters

Another factor influencing obesity-related health risks is the distribution of fat on your body. It is better to resemble a pear than an apple. Women tend to have more buttock and hip fat (pear shape) while men have more abdominal fat (apple shape). The major diseases and conditions related to being overweight are associated with increased abdominal fat.

Dieting

Dieting is difficult. Among those who succeed in losing weight, few manage to maintain that loss. Typically one third of the weight lost is regained within one year of the end of the diet, and almost all weight lost is regained within three to five years. Many regain additional pounds in addition to the weight they lose. A cycle of gain and loss referred to as yo-yo dieting can have serious negative consequences for health as well as self-esteem. For example, during weight loss you may lose both fat and lean tissue, but when weight is regained it may be primarily fat, leading to an increase in the percentage of body fat.

Losing weight can be dangerous

If you decide you need to lose weight then be sure to do it safely. Each year there is a new diet or diet pill to lose weight. Extreme diets can be dangerous, especially in older persons. Drastic reductions in food intake can result in vitamin and nutrient deficiencies. Diet pills should be the very last resort—they can cause death as well as serious damage to your health. For example, many individuals who took the diet pill combination Phen-Fen developed damage to their heart valves.

The basics of sound weight loss

A sound weight loss program has three components:

— Lower caloric intake (1,200-1,500 calories per day will minimize hunger and still allow weight loss)

— Increased physical activity (regular exercise is critical to a diet's success)

— A commitment to lifelong change in habits (regular exercise, enough sleep, stress reduction)

Diagnostic Evaluation of Nutritional Ill-health

The most helpful laboratory studies in assessing the nutritional status of a child are hematological studies and laboratory studies evaluating protein status. Hematological studies should include a complete blood count (CBC) with red blood cell indices and a peripheral smear. Measures of protein status include serum albumin, retinol-binding protein, prealbumin, transferrin, creatinine, and BUN.

In children who have a history of adequate food intake and signs/symptoms of malnutrition, focus on identifying the cause of malnutrition. Perform laboratory studies based on information from a complete history and physical examination.

Initial diagnostic laboratory studies include a CBC, sedimentation rate, serum electrolytes, and urinalysis and. culture. Stool specimens should be obtained if the child has a history of abnormal stools or stooling patterns or if the family uses an unreliable or questionable source of water.

Additional studies may focus on thyroid functions or sweat chloride tests, particularly if height velocity is abnormal. Further diagnostic studies should be determined as dictated by the history and physical examination.

Other Tests

- Practical nutritional assessment
- Complete history, including a detailed dietary history
- Growth measurements, including weight and length/height; head circumference in children younger than 3 years
- Complete physical examination
- Sensitive measures of nutritional status
- Height-for-age or weight-for-height measurements greater than 2 standard deviations below the mean for age
- Height-for-age or weight-for-height measurements more than 2 standard deviations less than the mean for age

— Height-for-age measurements less than 95% of expected value

— Weight-for-height measurements less than 90% of expected value

— Less than 5 cm/y of growth in children older than 2 years

— Body mass index (BMI)

Medical Care

Following evaluation of the child's nutritional status and identification of the underlying etiology of the malnutrition, dietary intervention in collaboration with a dietitian or other nutritional professional should be initiated. Children with edema must be assessed carefully for actual nutritional status because edema may mask the severity of malnutrition. Children with chronic malnutrition may require caloric intakes more than 120-150 kcal/kg/d to achieve appropriate weight gain. Additionally, any micronutrient deficiencies must be corrected for the child to attain appropriate growth and development. In mild-to-moderate cases of malnutrition, initial assessment and nutritional intervention may be done in the outpatient setting. A patient with malnutrition may require hospitalization based on the severity and instability of the clinical situation. Hospitalization of patients with suspected malnutrition secondary to neglect allows observation of the interactions between parent and child and documentation of actual intake and feeding difficulties.

Consultations

Any child at risk for nutritional deficiency should be referred to a registered dietitian or other nutritional professional for a complete nutritional assessment and dietary counseling. In the United States, children with poor nutrition secondary to inadequate intake should be referred to the appropriate social agencies to assist the family in obtaining resources and providing ongoing care for the child. Other subspecialty referrals are based on findings in the initial evaluation that may indicate a specific cause of inadequate nutrition other than inadequate food intake.

Balanced Diet

Protein, energy, and other nutrient requirements vary with age, sex, and activity levels.

Following careful assessment of the child's nutritional status, initiate nutritional intervention in collaboration with nutritional support personnel.

Children with chronic malnutrition may require caloric intakes in excess of 120-150 kcal/kg/d to achieve appropriate weight gain. The diet must include adequate amounts of protein and other macronutrients.

Any micronutrient deficiencies must be diagnosed and corrected to achieve adequate somatic growth and psychomotor development.

Further Outpatient Care

Monitor patients closely for growth and resolution of clinical signs and symptoms of malnutrition. Follow-up should be based on the severity of the illness, age of the patient, and the patient's initial response to intervention. Minimal intervals between visits should give the patient sufficient time to show a change in the measured parameter. For example, in infants beyond the newborn stage, the time needed to show an appreciable change in weight is 7 days. A 4-week interval is needed to document changes in length, and an 8-week interval is needed to document a change in height.

Deterrence/Prevention

Prevention of malnutrition in children starts with an emphasis on prenatal nutrition and good prenatal care. Health care providers should emphasize the importance of breastfeeding in the first year of life. Promotion of breastfeeding is particularly crucial in developing countries where safe alternatives to human milk are unavailable. In addition to the promotion of breastfeeding, health care providers should counsel parents on the appropriate introduction of nutritious supplemental foods. Health care providers should continue to provide age-appropriate nutritional counseling at every opportunity.

Programs addressing micronutrient supplementation and fortification have been successful at decreasing the incidence of specific micronutrient deficiencies (eg, iodine, vitamin D) in many countries. These programs should be promoted more in developing countries. Additional fortification programs should be developed to address other common nutritional deficiencies such as iron deficiency, which continues to be significant problem throughout the world. Improvement in hygiene practices and sanitation reduces the incidence of infectious diseases, which decreases the incidence of malnutrition in developing countries.

Prognosis

Children who have chronic malnutrition, particularly with onset at an early age, do not achieve their full growth potential or regain cognitive deficits. Although malnutrition is rare in the United States and other industrialized countries, half of childhood mortality in developing countries is secondary to malnutrition.

Adulteration of Food: Advesre Health Impacts

The adulteration of food was not uncommon in the nineteenth century; but it is important to look at this practice in the context of disease and death. What people relied on for strength and survival would no doubt have a say in their quality of life.

Many additives are used for aesthetic purposes as well as "practical" ones. The desire for consistent color and the need to stretch the food sold in order to gain greater profits led to many of these unhealthy practices. The adulteration of milk involved dilution with water and the addition of chalk. A recent survey report find that major cities between one quarter and one half of all samples [of milk] collected were contaminated. In 1860 it became an offence to adulterate milk. However, these rules were not strictly enforced and the fines for them were minimal in comparison to the profits that were gained by the additional sales this enhancement produced.

Food is the basic necessity of life. We toil day and night for two morsel of wholesome nutritive food. And if at the end of the day we are not sure of what we eat, than what are we toiling for? We may be eating a dangerous dye, sawdust, soap stone, industrial starch, Aluminum foil and believe it, even horse-dung! Inviting disease rather than good health. And what are the law enforcing authorities doing? Looking the other way, ignoring, sitting on files and being bought and bribed.

Milk that ever-enduring milk. For time immemorial it had had been the basic staple food right from our growing up stage, to when we have grown up. As a child we need it for growth and as a grown up we need it for replenishing our nutrition daily. Tired and bogged down, need something to rejuvenate, like a glass of milk. But even this has not been spared.

Common adulterant, addition of water, flour, or any other starchy material say industrial starch. Addition of water and extraction of fat is very common and not harmful. But what when the milk you drink is not milk at all? Rather combination of urea, liquid detergent, a little sugar, vegetable oil and water—a Synthetic Milk! Remember the case in Delhi, where the racket was busted a few years back and there was a lot of hue and cry in the media regarding the same. Think of all those children who may have had the synthetic milk, what havoc it must have created for their system physically.

Turmeric is the basic ingredient of Indian cooking. Any Indian dish is not complete without it. But before you buy your next quota of this "masala" be careful of what you are buying.

It may be adulterated with, Lead chromate, Metanil Yellow dye Or any starch based items like flour or rice powder or even industrial starch. Except flour or rice powder, all the other adulterants are health hazardous and cause irreparable damage to our system when eaten at regular intervals for a long period of time. Take for instance Lead chromate, it is one of the most toxic salts of lead. It can cause anemia, paralyses, mental retardation and brain damage in children and abortion in pregnant women. Metanil yellow dye which is another non-permissible toxic colorant, is used mostly to color *Besan* or gram flour, pulses, miscellaneous prepared foods namely sweetmeats like *ladoo, burfi, jelabi, dalmoth, papad,* etc. to get that attractive deep yellow color. Food grade colors are available in the market but being more costly, traders take advantage of the lackadaisical approach of the law enforcing authorities and substitute it with the said cheap and non-permissible dyes and colors.

While still on *"Masalas"* or spices, does one know what are the common adulterants, take for instance, for coriander powder or chili powder- sawdust, rice bran and sand. But wait! One cannot even imagine or fathom- horse-dung and cow-dung! This is not only unethical, from the business point of view, but a sin committed against the society at large. Any trader who is found resorting to such means of adulterations should be taken to task very strongly. People should try as far as possible to buy whole spices and grind them at home or purchase properly packed spices (with proper informative labeling) of standard F.P.O. I.S.I or AGMARK certified companies.

Has anyone ever given a thought why the puffed rice or any other white colored eatable looks so dazzling white and bright, and attractive on the show windows of a sweetmeat shop? Well they may have been treated by ultra marine blue a chemical dye which is a non-permissible and prohibited. And for that rich deep pink color (*Gulaabi*) Rhodamin-B is used-again a non-permissible colorant. This colorant has also proven to be carcinogenic.

Argemone seeds that grow as weeds in the mustered fields are mixed with mustered seeds and its oil is mixed with mustered oil. Just a trace amount is all right, but when added deliberately it causes serious health hazards and even death. Dropsy is a straight after effect of consumption of this oil. It may also cause swelling, irregular fever, low pulse rate, enlargement of the liver, respiratory distress which may lead to heart failure.

Adulteration of oil has become rampant, with a wide variety of oils available in the market, the consumer is not sure what combination of oils he gets when he buys it loose from the market. It is very harmful and hazardous to health when mixed with crude castor oil, industrial palmolein-oil, mineral oils etc. This is certainly a crime against humanity aimed at earning money at the cost of public health.

Ghee is adulterated to the extent of 80 to 85 percent with *Vanaspati* . In actuality it is *Vanaspati* flavored with 15 or 20 percent of ghee by special process. Even in the year 1935-36 when, six samples of so called pure ghee was collected it was found that they were adulterated with vegetable products made from groundnut, and other oils and the extent of adulteration was up to 80 percent.

Sand, dirt, earth, gritty matter, soap stone, common salt are added to flour, refined flour (*maida*), gram flour (*besan*), spices, sugar, tea-dust and coffee. And washing soda is added to table salt. In tea-dust one can even finds iron filings. And remember that lovely silver leaves used to decorate sweetmeats, *burfi*, and *pan*, you may be surprised what it is. It may be aluminum leave or foil, which is again very bad for health, causing a lot of physical complications.

Dried seeds of volatile oil are added to cloves, while mineral acids to vinegar, papaya seeds to black pepper. Aniseed or '*sauf*' that after food tit-bit, is dyed with malachite green dye for that nice green color. In food grains and whole spices extraneous matter like stalks, stems, and foreign seeds are added.

Castor oil which is often mixed in ground nut oil can cause abortion in cases of pregnant women. When the amount adulterated goes beyond 0.7 microgram per KG of body weight. He also adds that *Khesari Dal* which is often mixed in *Arhar Dal* can cause lower limb paralyses known as Lathyrism. Lathyrusativus species (*Khesari Dal*) has a toxic Amino acid known as Beta oxalyl amino alanine which is responsible for the above condition.

The consumer, to protect himself should avoid buying loose edible items from the markets, and go for tinned or packed items on which proper informative labels are displayed, which includes the date of manufacture and expiry as well. They should stress on products with F.P.O., I.S.I. or AGMARK certifications. These are the most commonly used certifications and at least gives the consumers third party guarantee of the product. The middle-class or the upper class can protect themselves by the above methods but what about the lower strata of the society, the laborers, the poor class who cannot afford to buy expensive packed items, who have to purchase only in small loose quantities daily due to economic constraints.

India do have the standards for food articles under Prevention of Food Adulteration Act, 1954. But what are the concerned law enforcing authorities or the said departments doing. Are they doing anything at all? 'Need' a social organization collected random samples from the market to get them tested. When they contacted the Pasteur Institute Shillong they were told that the results of the tests would take at least 40 days.

The maximum time required for each test is five to ten minutes which even a 10th grade science student can execute and perform. So the society made their own arrangements for testing the samples. What they found was very alarming. All the test results were positive. *Besan ladoos* had Metanil yellow dye. *Ghee* was adulterated with *Vanaspati, Chhena* (cottage cheese) had starchy material added to it. And the most important, remember the hue and cry for mustered oil? What a big scandal it was on the national level in our country a few years back? Almost all the loose samples collected gave strong traces and presence of argemone oil.

Only when mass death occurs do our authorities react and swing into action and start haphazardly banning items and articles and cause inconveniences to the public. Remember how difficult it was to get mustered oil when it was banned for a few days. But what about this slow poison we are consuming daily when the amount adulterated is not enough to kill us instantly, but slowly in the long process and over a long period of time. The consumer must be protected against any health hazards as well as fraud and adulterations. He should also be made capable of knowing the composition and the nutritive value of food he is buying through informative labeling And this can happen only when the concerned law enforcing departments are more vigilant and are really concerned for public health. But all the legislation cannot fully solve the problem of food contamination and adulterations unless the consumer himself becomes conscious of the hazards to health on such consumption and the law which are protecting him under such circumstances.

Consumers must be taught the provisions of the Food Laws and Regulations and how they are protected under the said Law. Only when, the people are aware of their rights to demand pure and nutritive food and start consumer movements, instead of bearing the brunt and suffering quietly and take to task any such unscrupulous traders or manufacturers by way of filling of PIL (Public Interest Litigation) in the courts or dragging them to consumer courts, will such serious social evils of food adulterations which has deep roots in our society can be uprooted and eradicated. If not for good, but then at least, it can be abated to a certain extent. Or else our future generations are certainly going to pay the price for our careless, negligent and easygoing approach to the whole issue.

5

Nutrition, Health, and Sports of Youth

The role and contribution of Youth are of vital importance in all countries. In a country like India where population is growing fast and the proportion of the young in the overall social and demographic profile is continuously increasing, the role of Youth becomes all the more significant. In India, youth as a distinct group comprises those men and women who are in the age group of 15 to 35 years. According to 1991 Census, there were approximately 340 million people in this age group, of which around 74 per cent lived in rural areas. The number rose to 380 million in 1997, which is expected to rise further to approximately 510 million by the year 2016.

The importance of the youth in national development has been a recurring theme in all Five Year Plans. The National Discipline Scheme introduced in the Second Plan continued in the Third Plan. The Fourth Plan gave special emphasis on the needs of the youth and on training leadership. Support was provided to voluntary organizations to participate in youth development programmes. Community Service was developed as an integral part of the curriculum for education, providing for instruction and training of all students enrolled in educational institutions.

During the Fifth Plan, the expansion and strengthening of National Service Scheme and Nehru Yuva Kendras (NYK) received emphasis. A National Service Volunteer Scheme (NSVS) was launched. In the Sixth Plan, an effort was made to have effective coordination of different programmes. A National Youth Policy was framed in the Seventh Five Year Plan and, accordingly, a Plan of Action was formulated in 1992. It was only in the Seventh Plan that the subject received a major boost, when the plan allocations were increased eight fold. The Ministry of Youth Affairs & Sports made major strides during the Eighth Plan period.

The number of Nehru Yuva Kendras went up from 398 to 499 and the number of youth clubs affiliated to Nehru Yuva Kendra Sangthan (NYKS) increased to 1,64,000 at the end of the Eighth Plan. The number of volunteers enrolled under National Service Scheme (NSS) also increased to 13.00 lakh. The Eighth Five Year Plan and the National Youth Policy had emphasized organizing the youth force for promotion of National & Cultural Integration, as well as fostering and developing interaction between youth from different parts of the country, especially the isolated border and tribal areas. It had also emphasized awareness-building and involvement of youth in social programmes relating to literacy, environment, health &family welfare, and community development.

Thrust Areas of Ninth Five Plan

For the Ninth Five Year Plan the thrust has been on harnessing Yuva Shakti, and the National Youth Policy emphasized the following:

1. Involving young persons in various community based National Building Activities;
2. Youth Empowerment & Gender Justice through inter-sectoral approach;
3. Providing special attention to education, training & employment, health, environment, sports, recreation and leisure, art & culture, science & technology, etc;
4. A new scheme called National Reconstruction Corps (NRC) has been introduced to involve youth volunteers in Nation Building Activities; and

5. Developing the interest of youth in development-oriented programmes.

Achievements

During the Ninth Five Year Plan, the activities of NYKS have been extended to provide more opportunity to rural youth. NYKS during the Ninth Five Year Plan has been able to extend its activities to a larger number of villages with offices in almost 500 districts. A number of new initiatives have been taken up by NYKS to involve rural youth by motivating them to organize themselves in youth clubs and self-help groups. Schemes like National Service Volunteer Scheme, Financial Assistance to Youth Clubs, Award to Outstanding Youth Clubs and Youth Development Centres have been successful in motivating young people towards development-oriented programmes.

The response of the students to the scheme of NSS has been quite encouraging. Starting with an enrolment of 40,000 students in 1969, the coverage of NSS students has increased to more than 17 lakhs during 2000-01. The scheme now covers all the States and the Universities of the country and has also made its presence felt at + 2 institutions in many States. Students, teachers, guardians, universities, colleges, schools and the people in general now realize the need and significance of NSS. Currently NSS is working on the theme which is quite relevant for the present day, i.e. "Youth for Healthy Society". Various other major programmes were undertaken by the NYKS during the Ninth Five Year Plan under the Swaran Jayanti Gram Swarozgar Yojana.

NYKS is implementing this project in collaboration with the Ministry of Rural Development, Government of India. The principal objective of the programme is to bring selected youth living below poverty line above the poverty line in 3 years.

Watershed Management Programmes are also being implemented by the NYKS. This project is being implemented in 800 villages of the 8 districts of Nalbari & Kamrup (Assam),

Gumta & Vaishali (Bihar), Jagatsingpur & Kalahandi (Orissa), Gwalior (M.P.) and Surguja (Chhatisgarh),respectively.

In addition to this, "assistance to disabled persons for purchase/fitment of aids and appliances - 100 old age day care centers" Project is being implemented in association with the Ministry of Social Justice &Empowerment in 100 districts where NYKS has active Youth Development Centres. Besides, several other programmes were undertaken by the NYKS such as 30 Gandhi Millennium Youth Peace Centres, Wild Life Watch Centres, National Youth Cooperative, UNDP - NYKS Youth Volunteers against Poverty Awards.

Approach for the Tenth Plan

At present, there are approximately 340 million people in the age group of 10-20 years in India, of which around 74 per cent lived in rural areas according to 1991 Census. Similarly, adolescent youth in the age group of 10-19 years account for 22.8 per cent of our population. This implies that about 230 million Indians are adolescents. It is proposed to target this segment of the youth population by way of some specific intervention strategies.

The thrust to include youth is to be made the focal point of National Planning and Development, Youth Empowerment, Gender Justice, Youth Health and Responsible Living.

The major thrust will be on involving youth in the process of National Planning and Development and making them the focal point of National Development. The major thrust will be to extend proper educational and training opportunities, to provide access to information in respect of employment opportunities including entrepreneurial guidance and financial credit. It is proposed to provide proper platforms for development of leadership qualities, democratic attitudes, open mindedness, insight, patriotism, role playing and self evaluation, etc. Youth will be involved in various policy making bodies.

The Ministry will play a pro-active and catalytic role in exploring and identifying employment opportunities for the youth of India by exploiting the vast natural and local resources of the country in a coordinated manner in collaboration with other Ministries/Departments of the Government so as to achieve the objective of optimal utilization of resources that have been invested in different schemes concerning youth.

The Ministry of Youth Affairs and Sports will play an active advocacy role to promote and propagate gender justice by making the youth themselves aware about their significance in the Indian context.

Youth activities will focus on providing quality health services and will ensure that youth have access to information in respect of reproduction, health, issues related toal coholism and drug addiction, etc.

It is necessary to address the problem of youth with special needs. For this purpose value based education will be imparted. These efforts will be enhanced by inculcating respect for elders and tolerance towards others' beliefs and religion, compassion for the poor and needy. Youth will be involved in protection and preservation of nature and will be provided opportunities for developing awareness in the field of cultural heritage and Indian history,

The adolescents need particular attention. A concentrated effort is needed to build a relatively stable place in society for adolescents, an effort which will have a profound influence in overcoming the barriers to the healthy development of young people.

Efforts will also be made to build a network of Government and NGO sectors for the development of youth.

Strategy for the Tenth Plan

The thrust of the youth programmes lies in a major expansion of the Nehru YuvaKendra and National Service Scheme with emphasis on vocational training and employment promotion. The Ministry of Youth Affairs & Sports will establish effective linkages both at the State and Central levels with all Departments and agencies involved in youth development work. The expansion of NYKS will be undertaken with a view to covering all the districts of the country and to mobilize and empower the youth by strengthening the youth club movement to cover at least 50% of the 6 lakh villages in India. The Youth Development Centres (YDCs) will be expanded to achieve the ultimate objective of one youth development centre in each of the 5000 blocks of the country. The YDCs are proposed to be made nodal centres of information for youth and, eventually, to become IT centres.

More youth clubs will be established, which have become the focal points of youth activities, so as to provide a platform for young people to raise issues concerning them

All segments of youth including rural youth should get opportunities to participate in various schemes like NCC/ NSS/Scouts & Guides and National Reconstruction Corps (NRC). The activities of NSS Network will be expanded to cover all degree colleges and +2 schools in states. Similarly, the activities of the National Reconstruction Corps (NRCs) are going to be expanding in 500 districts by the end of the Tenth Five Year Plan.

With a view to making the institute a truly National Centre for information, documentation, research and training concerning youth matters, the Rajiv Gandhi National Institute of Youth Development (RGNIYD) will be strengthened by providing additional resources in terms of manpower and material equipments.

The various schemes of the Department of Youth Affairs should be integrated ina manner that the focus is on harnessing energies of youth and encouraging them to participate in development activities.

The mass media needs to be mobilized more imaginatively and effectively for introducing sports culture in the country.

New Programmes

The term adolescent means to 'emerge or achieve identity' in the age group of 10 to 19 years. Adolescents have very special and distinct needs. It is essential to invest in adolescents, as they are the future of the country and require particular attention.

The most important issues regarding the adolescents are: i) Health, ii) Nutrition, iii) Education (Formal and Non Formal), iv) Vocation, v) Recreation and Sports, vi) Child Labour, vii) Children in difficult situations, viii) Alcohol and Drug Abuse, and ix) Role of Media in educating adolescents.

All adolescents should have access to education about family life, safe motherhood, reproductive health rights, sexuality, sexual responsibility, age at marriage, age at first pregnancy, family size, health care, hygiene, immunization, HIV/AIDS prevention, importance of education, particularly for girls, legal literacy, problems of drug and alcohol abuse, vocational opportunities and career planning. A scheme adolescents is proposed to be launched shortly.

The youth of the country seldom get a forum to debate issues concerning them and the nation at large, or to give expression to their abundant creative energies and exhibit their talents in fine Arts & Crafts. In view of this need, it is proposed to launch anew scheme for establishment of a National Youth Centre and similar centres in the states by providing outright capital grants by the Govt. of India.

Youth with Special Needs

There are certain sections of youth who suffer from various disabilities and handicaps both physical and mental. It is desirable that their facilities and services for them are coordinated, publicized and monitored by the Department of Youth Affairs as the nodal Department for all youth-related activities. It is therefore necessary to initiate a new scheme for counselling , career guidance, vocationalization of school education, life skill education, etc. for the welfare and development of the physically and mentally challenged. However, an in-depth study is needed before formulating effective programmes and action plans for this group.

The need and importance of physical education, games, sports and yoga are essential for health and physical fitness with a view to increasing individual productivity. The value of sports as a means to create potential for promoting social harmony and discipline is well recognized all over the globe. One of the basic issues in the field of education has been an acute realization of the fact that no education is complete without emphasis on sports and physical education.

Sports and Physical Education have been given due importance only since the year 1984 when a separate Department was created. It was only in 1999 that a separate Ministry was created. National College of Education and National Institute of Sports were established during the Second Five Year Plan and sports facilities like Stadia, Swimming Pools, and Open Air Theatre were constructed.

During the Third Five Year Plan, the National Coaching Scheme was introduced. The provisions under Physical Education, Games and Sports were increased during the Fourth Five Year Plan. During the Five Year Plan, coaching facilities for Sports were expanded. The Sixth Five Year Plan emphasized on spotting talent in different sports disciplines at a very young age for nurturing them to the level of excellence. Various facilities were created in different institutions for promising sports persons. During the Seventh Five Year Plan, emphasis was laid on Adventure Sports, development of infrastructure at the grassroot level. A National Sports Policy was formulated on the basis of which a Plan of action was formulated in 1992. Creation of a lot of sports infrastructure and laying of synthetic tracks and surfaces were undertaken during the Plan.

Many rural schools were assisted for development of play fields and sports equipment. Infrastructure facilities were also created in a number of colleges and universities. Talented schoolchildren in the age group 9 - 12 years were identified.

Special training was imparted to sports persons under Special Area Games (SAG) and Sports Project Development Area Centres (SPDA) schemes.

Thrust Areas of Ninth Year Plan

Thrust areas of the Ninth Plan are :

1. Development of excellence in sports, greater integration of scientific facilities and establishment of sound principles of sports physiology and sports medicine with requisite quality of manpower relevant to the training needs of the sports persons.
2. Enhancement of the competence and skills of coaches
3. Promotion of sports and physical education among girls and rural population.
4. Participation of State Governments in developing a comprehensive plan for development of sports.
5. Creation of sports infrastructure and making available such infrastructure to the public.
6. Promotion of people's participation in various sports activities.

Achievements

1. Creation of infrastructure and installation of synthetic playing surfaces and tracks have been undertaken during IX Five Year Plan.
2. Many National Federations, promising sports persons, were financially assisted; scholarships were also provided to sports persons and financial assistance was provided for promotion of rural sports during the Ninth Plan.
3. Performance of the Ninth Plan in terms of both Physical and financial targets have by and large been achieved.
4. Performance of Indian sports persons in the International arena has steadily improved.

Approach for the Tenth Plan

1. There is an immediate need to create a network of basic sports infrastructure throughout the country. More than creation, access to the infrastructure is of prime importance. Higher level of infrastructure is required to be created at district, state, and regional centers of SAI. For competitive sports, modern equipments and tools would be provided to enable the sports persons to compete in international events. During the Tenth Five Year Plan, training facilities at par with developed countries would be provided to sports persons. Dependency on foreign coaches will have to be phased out gradually and efforts will be made to upgrade coaching skills. There is an immediate need to carry out basic as well as applied research in sports related fields. Drug free environment is to be created by way of bringing effective checks to eliminate drug abuse in sports. Except for a few popular sports, which attract private sponsorship, a majority of sports activities are devoid of any opportunity for sports persons to adopt sport as a career. Hence, there is a need to have definite incentives for sports persons in the form of job reservation and awards.

2. Reservation, award and rehabilitation of outstanding sports persons will be taken up by providing job opportunities to them. During the Tenth Plan a multi-sectoral approach will be adopted for resource generation by tapping private and public sector resources to promote and develop sports activities in the country.

3. To achieve the above objectives, the Ministry has formulated a New National Sports Policy, which is awaiting final approval. The salient features of the policy are asunder:

   — Central Government would focus its attention on achieving excellence at the National & International Level while the State Governments will focus on broadbasing of sports.

- Working of federations/associations has to be more transparent, democratic, professional and accountable. Central Government will formulate a model organization structure as well as a set of guidelines and, if necessary, Central Legislation will be enacted.
- Very high priority will be given to promotion of sports in schools and rural areas. Village Panchayats and Youth and Sports clubs will be adequately mobilized for further promotion.
- Mass media will be mobilized for introducing a Sports culture in the country; disciplines will be prioritized on the basis of proven potential; popularity and performance and greater emphasis will be given to junior and sub-junior levels.
- Emphasis will be given to R&D.
- Annual Sports calendar of National Championships at various levels will be prepared and participation in International events by the Federations will be encouraged.
- Greater emphasis will be given to training, and development of sports scientists, judges, referees and umpires.

— Various corporate houses will be asked to adopt particular disciplines as well as sports persons for long term development. A National Sports Development Fund has been created with facility for 100 percent Income Tax exemption to the donors.

— Besides new initiatives, it has been decided to bring all the schemes that are in operation in the 9th Plan under the following six categories; (i) Schemes relating to infrastructure; (ii) Schemes relating to talent search and training; (iii) Schemes relating to events including holding of National/ International Sports Events; (iv) Schemes relating to awards; (v) Schemes relating to institutions; and (vi) Incentives for Promotion of Sports activities.

Strategy for the Tenth Plan

To make available adequate sports infrastructure to the public at large and in the vicinity, sports infrastructure in schools & colleges will be created. All urban bodies should earmark open spaces for playing fields whenever new colonies are being set up. A ban should be imposed on conversion of playing fields into housing/commercial complexes. Creation and development of sports infrastructure should be taken as an activity under NSS/NYK as well as through schemes of the Ministry of Rural Development; local bodies should also be involved in this area. Creation of Sports Infrastructure at District and Tehsil levels should be the responsibility of the State Governments. Higher level of sports infrastructure at District and State Headquarters should be created by the regional centre of Sports Authority of India for improving competitiveness. Modern equipments and tools will also be provided to enable the sports persons to enable them to compete in International Sports events.

Funding for broadbasing of sports should be done by the State Governments and the Government of India will augment the State Governments' efforts by extending financial assistance for the purpose.

Broadbasing of sports from village to state level by involving youth should be undertaken by organizing planned sports programme in educational institutions at community centres right from the village to state level. Sports Authority of India (SAI) should hold competitions for junior age groups at village, Taluka/ Mandal, District and State levels. Therefore, day to day involvement of youth in sports activities should be planned keeping in view the programmes at National level to enable the states to have adequate time to prepare the state teams for higher competitions where the youth can show their talents and bring medals to the state, besides enhancing their prospects for reaching higher levels in their career.

Sports activities particularly in rural areas should be selected keeping in view the facilities available. As far as possible the sports disciplines which do not require much equipment should be selected such as Kho Kho, Kabaddi, Volleyball, track and field events . For the promotion of sports in rural areas the Ministry of Rural Development should play an active role. Ministry should also extend assistance to the villages for the creation and maintenance of play fields and for providing sports equipment.

Where schools are located in villages, the implementation of day to day sports programme shall be entrusted to the Physical Education Teacher or any other classroom teacher. By participating in sports activities round the year, physical and mental fitness levels of the students will improve, which in turn, will contribute to the improvement of performance in sports as well as in academics. That will make the parents realize the importance and advantages of participation by their children insports activities.

Municipalities/Municipal Corporations should also contribute to the development of Sports in their areas. They should also ensure the maintenance of existing play fields/ stadia/swimming pools to involve a large number of youth in sports activities besides supplying the required quality sports equipment for day to day sports activities and for competitions.

Municipalities and Corporations should also organize competitions for all the Asian Games disciplines, particularly those disciplines which are popularly played at local and State level.

Government at Centre and State level should review the status of the Physical Education Colleges in the country and take appropriate measures to improve the Physical Education curriculum, the quality of teaching staff and the Infrastructure for practical classes.

In each state, Kendriya Vidyalayas and Navodaya Vidyalayas identified as sports schools should be allotted 2 to 3 disciplines to avoid overlapping and to cover all the Asian Games disciplines, as this competition will be our first target for winning more medals and to make a mark in the International Sports Arena.

Though the Inter University Competitions are being held every year in various disciplines, the Inter Collegiate programmes need to be strengthened. It should be made compulsory for all the colleges to organize Inter College Competitions and to participate in the university competitions. The Inter University Programme should be made more attractive in order to inspire the University students to take part in sports activities and represent their colleges at University level and then the University in Inter-University Competitions. The strengthening of the University Sports Programme would contribute to improve the performance of National Teams.

There is another important area that needs attention. The talented boys and girls at various levels should be provided with standard quality sports equipment for day to day training and competitive opportunities to improve their performance. Care should be taken to avoid injuries due to faulty equipment. The Domestic Sports Industry should be encouraged by giving them incentives for manufacturing International Standard Equipment. Till that time, good quality equipment needs to be imported for training as well as for competitions.

There is an immediate need to create a network of basic sports infrastructure throughout the country starting with schools/colleges, etc. Therefore, it is necessary to insist on proper maintenance and utilization of infrastructure/synthetic tracks. A tie up with sports hostels and State Level Training Centers may be worked out for ensuring better utilization of these facilities.

The procedures relating to identification of disciplines, selection and preparation of Indian sports persons/sports teams, identification of national coaches, selection of sports persons for inclusion in coaching camps, venues of coaching camps, designing of a battery of physical fitness/medical/skill tests during coaching camps and additional facilities for substantive coaching camps would all be taken into account for preparing an implementable plan for building up and enhancing medal winning capabilities of Indian sports persons.

Besides the concerned federations and the State Governments, private and public sector organizations would also have to be fully involved with the formulation and implementation of the Plan. However, such a short-term Plan must have a long-term perspective of broadbasing sports with a view to achieving physical fitness for all and excellence in sports through talent spotting and nurturing.

There is an imperative need for creation of desired sports climate in the country and consciousness in every citizen to be physically fit and to participate in games and sports. This requires the creation of sports infrastructure in a planned manner, more efficient use of available sports infrastructure and coaching facilities with promction activities like 'Bhartiyam'.

The envisioning of a pyramidal structure for sports promotion is required, beginning with primary and secondary schools and ending at college level. For development of resource potential, an adequate number of physical education teachers are required. In addition to the play fields at the school stage and necessary' encouraging' environment for willing students to make further progress, there is a need to provide adequate support to the SAG and NSTC schemes, which provide opportunities to potential sports persons in tribal, remote and rural areas for getting them trained in selected disciplines. A related aspect is the need to have separate infrastructure for sports institutions. In India, we have made a beginning in this regard by developing sports infrastructure in the regional and other centers of SAI.

For excellence in sports, the back-up of improved technology is necessary. Specific efforts should be made for tapping indigenous potential available for swimming in coastal areas and archery in tribal areas.

Sports schools should be set up in states in collaboration with private sector by providing them with attractive incentives.

Sports and physical education should be integrated effectively in the educational curriculum.

A policy needs to be evolved for promoting the participation of NGOs and industrial houses in sports.

Ministry of Youth Affairs and Sports should formulate a special scheme for the promotion of sports and games for the disabled persons.

Financial Allocations for the Tenth Plan

For the Ninth Five Year Plan, Ministry of Youth Affairs & Sports has been allocated an amount of Rs.826.09 crore (Rs.352.24 crore for Youth Development Programmes, Rs.472.61 crore for Sports Development and Rs.1.24 crore for Secretariat Social Services). For the Tenth Five Year Plan, an amount of Rs.3287.51 crore (Rs.1534.45 crore for Youth Programmes, Rs.1750.58 crore for Sports Programmes and Rs.2.48 crore for Secretariat Social Services) has been suggested by the Working Group on Youth Affairs & Sports. Outlays proposed by the Working Group for the Tenth Five Year Plan is four times greater than the approved outlay of Ninth Five Year Plan. The budgetary support that could be provided by the Planning Commission for Youth Affairs & Sports will depend on the total size of the budgetary support allocated by the Ministry of Finance for the Plan, and further on the inter-sectoral priorities fixed by the Planning Commission for the Plan as a whole.

The Steering Committee also wanted the Department to prioritize the schemes, both the continuing ones and the new schemes proposed for the Tenth Plan. The Ministry was also requested to tap resources of both private and public sector for promotion of sports in the country. The new initiatives proposed in the Tenth Plan include promotion of Sports and tourism with a focus on recreational and adventure Sports, and the settingup of sports academies in the States.

Nutrition and Health of School-Age Children

The success of child survival programmes and the expansion of basic education coverage have resulted in a greater number of children reaching school age with a higher proportion actually attending primary school. However, there is increasing evidence, with resulting international concern, that the high level of nutritional deprivation combined with the heavy burden of disease in this age group has negative consequences for a child's long term overall development. This has prompted an increased focus on the diverse needs of the school-age child.

An understanding and awareness of the heavy burden of malnutrition and disease among school-age children is growing although until recently there have been relatively few large scale surveys that document levels of morbidity in any detail. While a better picture of the health and nutrition status of this age group is being built, the true extent of the burden of ill health and malnutrition is still not fully known.

The main nutritional problems facing the school-age child include stunting, underweight, anaemia and iodine deficiency and, on the basis of information from recent surveys, vitamin A deficiency. In countries experiencing the 'nutrition transition', overweight and obesity are increasing problems in the school-age child. The main health problems facing school-age children are malaria, helminth infections, diarrhoeal diseases, respiratory infections and the direct and indirect effects of HIV/AIDS. Much of the disease burden derives from the poor environmental conditions in which children live including exposure to biological, chemical and physical hazards in the environment and a lack of resources essential for human health.

Malnutrition

Malnutrition refers to disorders resulting from an inadequate diet or from failure to absorb or assimilate dietary elements. Stunting (low height-for-age) is a physical indicator of chronic or long term malnutrition and is often linked to poor mental development. Stunting is a cumulative process of poor growth that primarily occurs before the age of three years and is not easily reversed. This infers that these first years of life provide a window of opportunity for effective nutritional programming. Underweight (low weight-for-age) is an indicator of both chronic and acute undernutrition. Wasting (low weight-for-height) is an indicator of acute undernutrition. Few representative data are available on the levels of malnutrition in school-age children, however, the available data on school-age children follow the regional pattern of the more extensive representative data from surveys of preschool children.

Preschool Children

The prevalence of stunting, underweight and wasting varies by region and subregion throughout low income countries. The Africa region has the highest estimated prevalence of stunting (20.2-48.1%) and has the lowest rate of improvement. In East Africa sub-region, rates of stunting are increasing. The prevalence of stunting in Asia (32.8-43.7%) is also high, particularly in South Central Asia, although rates of stunting continue to improve throughout this region.

In Latin America and the Caribbean, the prevalence of stunting is significantly lower (9.3-24%) than the other two regions and is improving, except in the Central America sub-region. For preschool children, the prevalence of underweight and wasting follow similar regional patterns to the prevalence of stunting. Estimates for prevalence of underweight pre-school children in different regions of Africa in the year 2000 range from 14 to 36.5% underweight; Asia 28.9 to 43.6% and Latin America and the Caribbean 3.2 to 15.4%. Although estimates of prevalence of wasting are not available for all sub-regions, overall estimates for wasting in preschool children by region are available for 1995: Africa 9.6%, Asia 10.4% and Latin America and the Caribbean 2.9%.

School Children

Stunting is widely believed to occur mainly in early childhood (mostly by three years of age), and through a cumulative process. Children stunted at school-age are likely to have been exposed to poor nutrition since early childhood and that the degree of stunting tends to increase throughout the school-age years. However, children can exhibit catchup growth if their environment improves. This suggests that interventions in school-age children can supplement efforts in the preschool years to reduce levels of stunting and related effects on children's health and education.

Underweight among school-age children, like stunting, can reflect a broad range of insults such as prenatal undernutrition, deficiencies of macro- and micronutrients, infection and, possibly, inadequate attention by caregivers. Wasting, which reflects acute malnutrition, is not as common as either stunting or underweight in school-age children. Nevertheless, wasting rates can change rapidly in situations of acute food crisis, with school-age children, adolescents in particular, becoming severely malnourished in such situations.

Recent studies on school-age children have shed new information on stunting, wasting and underweight for this age group:

— one of the largest studies of anthropometric status of rural school children in low income countries (Ghana, Tanzania, Indonesia, Vietnam and India) found the overall prevalence of stunting and underweight to be high in all five countries, ranging from 48 to 56% for stunting and from 34 to 62% for underweight. Second, in all countries there was a trend for scores for height-for-age and weight-for-age to decrease with age, thus as children got older they became progressively shorter relative to the reference population. Third, the boys in most countries tended to be more stunted than girls and in all countries boys were more underweight than girls

— in height and weight of school-age children on Pemba Island, Zanzibar showed the prevalence of stunting increased with age (14% prevalence in seven year olds increasing to 83% in 13 year olds) and peaked in girls at age 12 then declined when they entered their pubertal growth spurt. In boys, however, the prevalence of stunting rose steadily up to age 13 years and then slowly declined. Boys accumulated a height deficit of 11.9cm and girls a height deficit of 8.5cm compared to the reference population

— the nutritional status of adolescent boys and girls in Bangladesh found that 67% of adolescents were thin (BMI< 5th percentile of WHO reference) and 48% were stunted (defined as height-for-age <5th percentile of the NCHS and WHO reference data). Whereas, thinness was found to decline in prevalence with age from 95% at age 10 years to 12% at age 17 years, the prevalence of stunting increased from 34% at age ten years to 65% at age 17 years. Stunting was also found to increase with age in a second study with younger girls reported to have a prevalence of just 2% stunting while 16% of older girls were stunted

— in Brazil of the gender differences in growth of school-age children suffering from helminth infections found that 21% of school-age children were stunted and 13% were underweight. Both indices of nutritional status worsened as the study population got older, particularly for boys. The later onset of puberty and the growth-spurt in boys was controlled for in the growth data analysis, but boys remained significantly more malnourished than girls.

— in school-age children in Bangladesh, diarrhoea was found to retard weight gain and slow linear growth, although respiratory infections did not have the same effect

— an impoverished rural area of Guatemala that had recently benefited from a poverty alleviation programme, identified sanitation and housing conditions as risk factors for growth faltering in school-age children. Adult women's body mass index was also identified as a risk factor for stunting in school-age children three recent studies from Chile also link growth deficits in school-age children to socioeconomic conditions:

— in indigenous Chilean school children, improved social conditions were related to improved growth, but this was not observed among the nonindigenous school children

— the risk factors of short stature among Chilean children entering school, reports similar risk factors associated with short stature (and poverty) independent of parents' heights, suggesting that genetic factors have limited impact on height at this age. The authors conclude that in countries similar to Chile, in order to decrease the prevalence of growth deficits, reducing poverty and its consequences is critical

— Chile concluded that the higher prevalence of stunting among an indigenous population of Mapuche school children was not genetic, but reflected socioeconomic conditions. The study found no significant differences in growth deficits among school children of Mapuche ancestry compared to non- Mapuche ancestry within poverty levels.

— the severity and prevalence of stunting and underweight have been found to increase with age, with older children diverging further from the reference medians for height until puberty. The evidence suggests that boys are more likely to be stunted and underweight than girls, and in some countries, more likely to be wasted than girls. This may be due to a bias in the school population. It is also suggested that it could reflect delayed onset of puberty

— it appears that although children (of both sexes) show evidence of growth into late adolescence, full 'catch-up' growth is not occurring and linear growth retardation persists throughout the school years. Nonintervention studies of catch-up growth in children show moderate levels of improvement, with 25-32% of the children stunted at age 2 years no longer stunted by school-age or pre-adolescence

— comparing preschool stunting to stunting in adolescence, stunted girls exhibited a significant delay in sexual maturation and showed evidence of catch-up growth between the ages of five and 17 years. The girls' delay in sexual maturity demonstrates that stunted children of both sexes have the possibility of catch-up growth after age 17 years. The stunted girls on average had a 1.6 year delay in menarche compared to the tallest girls

— rural Bangladesh, menarche was associated with better nutritional status as indicated by significantly higher mean heights (in menstruating girls ages 11-14 years) and weights (in menstruating girls ages 13-15 years) compared to non-menstruating girls of the same ages

— evidence suggests that in adolescence, children in deprived environments grow as much, or more than the NCHS reference population and that during the childhood period, tremendous variation in growth exists between populations

— in Chile, a country undergoing the 'nutrition transition', height deficits have been compared between children entering first grade in 1987, 1990, 1993 and 1996. Overall, height deficits have declined in both boys (from 10.6% in 1987 to 7.3% in 1996) and girls (from 7% in 1987 to 5% in 1996), although the overall height deficit in boys was found to be greater than for girls in each period studied. Stunting was found to increase with age: 2.2% of 5-6 year olds were stunted compared to 13.1% in children over 8 years old; and

— rather large height deficits can accumulate during the relatively long childhood period of about 8 years. Whilst growth can be improved during the childhood period, growth improvements observed in studies of one year or less duration have been disappointing. Longer-term interventions need to be conducted to determine if gains in growth can be sustained long enough to become significant.

From the mid-90s several studies have focused on the health status on out-of-school children.

— in Ghana compared the health of enrolled and non-enrolled children in primary school and showed that there were considerable differences between enrolled and non-enrolled children. Nonenrolled children of both sexes were significantly smaller in height than enrolled children of the same age range. Just over half (51%) of children aged six to seven years who were not enrolled in primary school were stunted in comparison with only 19% who were enrolled in school. It is likely that many of the chronic health problems encountered in the six to seven year old children studied are the product of disease and poor nutrition before they enrolled in school.

Important questions are raised from these studies that reflect the need for more information on the patterns and determinants of growth in this age group. First, it is important to identify whether the height deficits accrued during the primary school years are made up through longer pubertal growth and at what stage boys and girls stop growing in height. Second, the functional implications of linear growth retardation in school-age children needs to be more clearly understood. Third, the question as to what extent schoolage stunting is preventable through school-based interventions needs to be addressed.

Impact of Undernutrition on Children's Education

The studies of the effect of undernutrition on cognitive ability although not entirely conclusive, indicate that chronic undernutrition is associated with lower achievement levels in school children. Recent studies have found:

— that severe stunting in the first two years of life is strongly associated with lower test scores in school-age children (age 8-11). However, deficits in children's scores were smaller at older ages, suggesting that adverse effects may decline over time. In addition, lower test scores were related to later enrollment, increased absenteeism and repetition of school years among stunted children. These findings' indicate that stunted and nonstunted children can benefit similarly from education

— a negative association between indicators of chronic malnutrition and language and mathematics test scores in a cross sectional study of 3,055 Vietnamese school children when indices of malnutrition to educational test scores were compared; and

— short stature has been associated to late enrollment for primary school children in Tanzania and Ghana.

Micronutrient Deficiencies

Nutritional anaemia, particularly deficiencies of iron, iodine, and vitamin A are major problems for school-age children in low income countries. It has been shown that such deficiencies can negatively impact on growth, increase susceptibility to infection and also impair the mental development and learning ability of school children.

Iron Deficiency and Anaemia

Iron deficiency (ID) is the most common nutritional disorder in the world and is estimated to affect more than 2b people of whom 1.2b suffer from iron deficiency anaemia (IDA). Insufficient intake of iron rich foods is the major cause of ID. It can also be caused by parasitic infections (particularly hookworm and malaria) and deficiencies of other nutrients.

There is little evidence to suggest any recent decrease in the prevalence of anaemia. It is estimated that 53% or 210m school-age children suffer from IDA. The highest prevalence is reported in Asia (58.4%) followed by Africa (49.8%). Recent studies and surveys have tried to capture the prevalence of IDA in school children:

— around 14,000 rural school children in Africa and Asia, the prevalence of IDA was more than 40%in five African countries (Mali, Tanzania, Mozambique, Ghana, and Malawi) amongst children aged 7-11 years and in four African countries amongst children aged 12-14 years. In the two Asian countries studied, the overall prevalence of IDA was found to be considerably lower than in Africa (around 12% in Vietnam and 28% in Indonesia among 7-11 year olds). Children aged 7-11 years were found to have lower mean haemoglobin concentrations, while IDA was found to be more common in the older age group. Girls were also found to have lower haemoglobin concentrations than boys, although the overall prevalence of IDA was higher in boys, particularly in the 12-13 year age group. An association between late enrollment in school, as compared to enrolling closer to the correct age, and a higher prevalence of anaemia was also found

— nearly 2,998 children ages 8-9 and 12-13 years in Ghana and Tanzania revealed that 77% of children in Tanzania and 41% of children in Ghana were suffering from IDA

— 1,210 primary school girls aged 7-14, in Riyadh, Saudia Arabia, an anaemia level of 55.4% was found. The highest level (71.4%) was found among 14 year-old girls

— adolescent males and females in Bangladesh, extremely high levels of anaemia were identified in both females (98%) and males (94%). At age 17, 100% of females were anaemic, and

— in 6,486 adolescent students (12-15 years) in East Java, Indonesia, anaemia levels of over 25% in girls, 24% in pre-pubertal boys and 12% in pubertal boys were detected. Higher levels of anaemia were found among adolescents of lower socioeconomic status.

There is substantial evidence that IDA in children is associated with decreased physical development, impaired immune function, poor growth and increased fatigue. IDA also affects cognitive function and school achievement.

— in Thailand, large differences were found between school children with anaemia and/or iron deficiency and iron replete children in their performance on a Thai language test and a test of general reasoning ability, yet not in arithmetic scores

— Soemantri found smaller differences between Indonesian school children with IDA and iron replete children in their performance on a range of school exams, although the children did not differ in a test of concentration. Both exam performance and concentration was improved by iron supplementation

— iron supplementation improved the performance of Indian school children on tests of memory and visual/ motor coordination.

Impact of Supplementation on INA

The main focus of IDA reduction programmes has been young children and women of reproductive age. Recent studies have emphasized the high prevalence of iron deficiency and anaemia in school-age children. This has resulted in an increased programmatic response for this age.

However, there is conflicting evidence concerning the beneficial effect of iron supplementation on growth in children. Some studies have shown that daily supplementation improves growth and appetite, while others have not found any beneficial growth response:

— results from one study indicate that four months of daily supplementation with 3 mg ferrous sulphate per kilogram of body weight of non-iron replete, nonanaemic children results in decreased weight gains

— pre-school and school children concludes that iron supplementation has significant impact on the linear growth in anaemic children

— the effects of providing weekly doses of 400 mg of ferrous sulphate for three months on the iron status and growth of adolescent schoolgirls in Tanzania was conducted. Weekly iron supplementation was found to result in a significant increase in serum ferritin (but not haemoglobin) and a significant increase in weight gain compared to adolescents given a placebo. No gain in height was found

— in a randomized controlled trial of non-anaemic school-age children receiving 3mg ferrous sulphate per kg bodyweight or a placebo, weekly for 18 weeks, the treatment group did not show any significant change in haemoglobin, however the control group showed a significant decrease in haemoglobin concentrations.

Changes in weight were not significantly different between the treatment and control groups. In recent years, a number of studies have suggested that weekly iron supplementation is as effective as daily supplementation in raising haemoglobin levels, however, there is a still a need to further assess the effectiveness of weekly supplements under programme conditions to ensure that compliance is achieved.

— in Bolivia suggest that iron supplementation (3-4mg/kg ferrous sulphate) for five days per week is as effective as weekly supplementation over the course of 16 weeks

— in 60 non-formal schools in Mali found that supplementation with 65mg iron and 250 μg folic acid weekly for 10 weeks improved haemoglobin concentration by 3.9 g/L in comparison with a placebo group. All children were given deworming treatment and vitamin A supplements prior to the trial

— Africa that has examined the impact of weekly supplementation with 400mg of ferrous sulphate for four months on the iron status and growth of adolescent schoolgirls found a significant increase (>50%) in serum ferritin levels in the group receiving iron supplements

— reducing anaemia in adolescent schoolgirls in Peru tested both daily and intermittent iron supplementation (60mg of ferrous sulphate) over a 17 week period. It was found that while both supplementation schedules resulted in improved iron status, daily supplementation resulted in the greatest increase in haemoglobin concentration and significantly reduced the prevalence of anaemia

— an experimental community trial was conducted to observe the effect of a communication programme on compliance with weekly iron supplementation (65 mg elemental iron + 250 µg folic acid) in urban Tanzanian adolescent schoolgirls. A total of 237 girls, aged 14-17 were randomly recruited from five schools. Girls in schools 1 and 2 received iron and folic acid tablets weekly for eight weeks and weekly communication sessions, school 3 received the same supplement without the communication sessions and schools 4 and 5 served as the control schools. In the group receiving supplementation and communication, the prevalence of anaemia decreased significantly.

The prevalence of anaemia did not change significantly in schools 3 and 4 but increased significantly in school 5. The observed compliance in the schools receiving the communication sessions was 75 and 94% compared to 50% in the school without the communication sessions. These results suggest communication strategies can influence compliance with iron supplements and thus help to reduce anaemia in adolescents; and

— Indonesia and Malaysia have demonstrated improvements in the iron stores of adolescent schoolgirls supplemented once weekly. In the Indonesian study, the group who received retinol along with the iron supplement benefited most in terms of increased iron stores.

Iodine Efficiency and Iodine Deficiency Disorders (IDD):

Iodine deficiency affects an estimated 1.6b people worldwide and estimated 60m school-age children. The consequences of iodine deficiency include severe mental retardation, goitre (a condition involving the enlargement of the thyroid gland and a disruption of normal thyroid production), hypothyroidism, abortion, stillbirths and low birthweight and mild forms of motor and cognitive deficits. Recent studies in school-age children have found very high levels of goitre and iodine deficiency. School-age children are often the target population of IDD assessments because of their physiological vulnerability and their accessibility.

— IDD in school children have been carried out in Egypt, Swaziland and South Africa. Overall prevalence rates of between 35 and 70% have been found indicating a severe public health problem in each of areas studied.

— in Calcutta, India, after having implemented a universal iodized salt programme for several years, a monitoring survey reported 23% of male school children and 32% of female school were moderately to severely iodine deficient.

Children's Mental Development and Education

Iodine deficiency is the leading cause of preventable intellectual impairment worldwide. A number of studies comparing children living in iodine-deficient areas with those living in iodine sufficient areas have found that the iodine deficient children have poorer levels of cognitive development and school achievement.

— over the past 30 years, have found that school-age children living in iodine-deficient areas have lower IQs and poorer cognitive and motor function than school-age children living in iodine-sufficient areas

- in school-age children suffering from mild and moderate iodine deficiency in Bangladesh, it was found that hypothyroid children performed worse than normal children in reading and spelling.
- the association between hypothyroidism and cognitive and motor function and school achievement in Bangladeshi school-age children found that the hypothyroid children performed worse in reading and spelling than non-hypothyroid children. These differences were observed after controlling for biological, socio-cultural and socio-economic conditions. In addition it was found that stimulation and the availability of materials were also significantly associated with improved reading, spelling and mathematics. Children suffer a range of disadvantages in addition to iodine deficiency and if they are to benefit fully from education, a comprehensive approach to their health and nutrition problems is needed; and
- in Benin, a randomized control trial was implemented on an iodine-deficient population of 196 school children. Due to the availability of iodized salt to the study population during the intervention, participant results were split post hoc based on improved iodine status measured in urine samples. Results indicate that children with improvements in urinary iodine status (from capsules or iodized salt) had significantly better test scores, particularly on tests of abstract reasoning and verbal fluency compared to children without improvements in iodine status. As the tests included time limits for response, these findings may indicate an improvement in the level and or speed of task performance. These results may indicate a "catchup" effect as well. The group of children whose urinary iodine concentrations were unchanged during the intervention showed less progress even though their iodine status was, on average, better than the improved group both initially and at the end of the study. Universal iodization of salt is seen as the permanent and sustainable solution to the global IDD

problem. Iodization of salt is the preferred approach for supplementation in iodine deficient populations. It is now mandatory for manufactured salt to be iodized in most countries, however, this does not guarantee the elimination or reduction of IDD. In many countries a persistence of goitre in school children is being observed despite near universal iodized salt consumption.

In areas where iodized salt is not available and where the prompt correction of IDD is urgent, iodized oil can be administered to school children inexpensively and simply, maintaining iodine levels for a period of twelve months.

— in Guatemala where the purchase of iodized salt has been problematic, IDD education through schools has been piloted. It was found that a participatory education module appeared to result in an increase in the purchase of iodized salt at the household level

— in South Africa, where mandatory iodization of salt was introduced in 1995, a study of the effects on school children in an endemically goitrous area after one year found that iodine deficiency was virtually eradicated.

The overall goitre rate, however, did not decline

— in China, a randomized clinical trial was implemented comparing iodine interventions in 205 school children aged 8-10 with low to moderate levels of iodine deficiency. Group A was provided iodized salt with an iodine concentration of 25 ppm; groups B and C purchased iodized salt from the market, while group C was provided with an iodized oil capsules at the beginning of the study. The salt iodine level for group A was stable, however for group B and C the salt iodine levels ranged from 13-47 ppm. The children in Groups A and C responded more quickly than group B, with a higher percentage decline in iodine deficiency, as measured in abnormal thyroid volumes; and

— in a recent trial conducted in an area of endemic goitre, the response of oral iodine supplementation in anaemic and non-anaemic goitrous children was compared. In the children with iron deficiency anaemia their response to oral iodine was impaired.

Multiple Micronutrient Deficiencies

Single micronutrient deficiencies seldom occur in isolation, but instead, interact and tend to cluster. For example, iron deficiency and Vitamin A Deficiency (VAD) often coexist in the same populations. Providing vitamin A supplementation can both improve vitamin A status, as well as, iron metabolism in deficient populations. Further, vitamin A food fortification programmes produce similar results.

School-age children, like most populations in low income countries, suffer from multiple micronutrient deficiencies. Data are not available on the extent of the problem in school-age children. However, inference can be made from data on pre-school children; 13 to 27% of pre-school school children are estimated to have two or more micronutrient deficiencies suggesting that 100m pre-school children are affected. Given the frequent overlap and clustering of micronutrient deficiencies, multiple micronutrient supplementation or fortified foods may be a cost-effective strategy to address nutrient deficiencies in school-age children, in addition to synergistic effects between certain micronutrients.

— in China, children supplemented with zinc and other micronutrients had the largest improvements in growth and cognitive function; growth improved with micronutrient supplementation, but showed little change with only zinc supplementation. These results are consistent with other studies and suggest that deficiencies of other micronutrients can suppress the growth response after zinc repletion

— the relationship between vitamin A, iron status and helminth infection among Bangladeshi school children, children with low serum retinol levels had significantly lower ferritin and haemoglobin levels that those with higher serum retinol levels

— in a randomized double-blind control trial with 830 primary school children from Tanzania, the odds of stunting were significantly reduced by provision of a micronutrient-fortified beverage. Anaemia was reduced nearly by half in the intervention group as well. The children drank one serving of the beverage, fortified with 30-120% of the RDA for several micronutrients for six months on each attended school day.

— in Tanzania, a randomized controlled trial of the effects of dietary supplements on anaemia, and on the weight and height of 136 anaemic school children from low socio-economic backgrounds was conducted. The supplements were administered for three months in local corn meals. Although vitamin A supplementation increased haemoglobin levels and growth parameters significantly, the group of children who received the combined vitamin A and iron supplements had the greatest improvements compared with the placebo group in all indicators. Vitamin A and iron supplementation have a role in the prevention of IDA and growth retardation

— a randomized, double-blind, controlled study of the effects of dietary supplements on anaemia in teenagers was conducted in urban Bangladesh. Participants were provided weekly supplements for 12 weeks. Compared with the placebo, the iron, folic acid and vitamin A supplement reduced anaemia by 92%, iron deficiency by 90% and vitamin A deficiency by 76%. For young women not deficient in vitamin A, there was not a significant difference in the response of haemoglobin to iron than to iron plus vitamin A. Those with the lowest baseline haemoglobin had the greatest increase in haemoglobin

— giving micronutrient deficient school children in South Africa biscuits fortified with iron, iodine and beta-carotene has been shown to significantly improve their micronutrient status. The prevalence of low serum retinol concentrations decreased from 39.1% to 12.2 %, anaemia declined from 27.8% to 13.9% and low urinary iodine concentrations declined from 97.5% to 5.4%. The biscuit was given in the morning for a period of 215 days at a cost of just US$0.7 per child, per school year

— in 66 school children (aged 10- 12) in India, those identified as deficient in iron and vitamin A were fed biscuits made with cauliflower leaf powder (a source of iron and vitamin A) for a period of four months. After the intervention, the experimental group had significantly higher haemoglobin and serum retinol levels. Initially 27.27% of children in the experimental group had normal nutritional status compared to 42.42% post intervention; and

— in a randomized control trial of the effect of antihelminthic treatment and micronutrient fortification in 579 South African school children aged 8-10 years, children were randomly allocated into six study groups, half who received anti-helminthic treatment at baseline. Each of the two groups were further divided into three groups and given biscuits (for 16 weeks) either unfortified, fortified with iron, or fortified with iron and vitamin A. There was a significant treatment effect of vitamin A on serum retinol levels, as well as, a suggested additive effect between vitamin A fortification and deworming, i.e. vitamin A supplementation with deworming had a greater effect on vitamin A status than vitamin A fortification alone. At baseline 34.7% of the children were vitamin A deficient and 15.5% were anaemic. Significant cognitive treatment effects were not found in either of the groups that received biscuits fortified with multiple micronutrients.

The impact of this intervention may have been limited by its short duration (16 weeks), low burden of micronutrient deficiency and low prevalence of stunting in the study population.

Overweight and Obesity

Overweight and obesity is becoming increasingly prevalent in low income countries where improvements in socioeconomic conditions and rapid urbanization are causing a 'nutrition transition'. A rapid shift in the composition of diet (higher fat and lower carbohydrate), reduced activity patterns and a subsequent shift in body composition characterize this transition. Countries undergoing a 'nutrition transition' have high levels of stunting, which is believed to be a risk factor for obesity. This may be explained by the relationship of stunting to undernutrition. Evidence from animal and human studies suggests that with malnutrition in utero and in early life, endocrine development may be affected, resulting in hormonal alterations and a predisposition to metabolic disorders and obesity. It is suggested that the increased risk of obesity among stunted children will lead to considerable problems with obesity in children in low income countries over the coming decades.

Although there is a growing body of data on obesity and overweight in this age group, few data are available on the true extent of overweight among school-age children in low income countries. Nationally representative data are lacking and few countries have repeated surveys, thus trend data are limited. Furthermore, there are methodological concerns, the use and interpretation of weight-for-height indices based on children from the US has been questioned in populations with significant levels of stunting.

In 1995, an estimated 17.6m children in the low income countries were overweight. The overall prevalence of overweight in the pre-school population is low, at 3.3%. Available data suggest that the problem of obesity begins in preschool children, becoming more evident among school-age children. In Sub- Saharan Africa and in South Asia obesity is rare. However, in the more developed countries of Latin America, the Middle East, Central Eastern Europe, the Commonwealth Independent States and North Africa, obesity is as prevalent as in the United States. Northern Africa and

Central America, areas undergoing rapid nutrition transitions, have both problems of stunting and overweight among children. In school-age children, the following has been observed:

— in Chile, 20.7% of school-age children were reported to be overweight and 13.5% obese in 1995

— school-age children (and pre-schoolage) in four countries undergoing the nutrition transition (Russia, China, Brazil and South Africa) found that the prevalence of child overweight ranged from 10.5% to 25.6% (weight-for-height at or above the 85 percentile). Boys in Russia have an overweight prevalence comparable with boys in the US (11.8% >95 percentile). Stunting is also common in these countries affecting between 9% and 30% of all children and a significant association was found between stunting and overweight status in all four countries

– from China, urban-rural combined data comparing the level of overweight school children from 1991 to 1995 indicate increases of 6 to 9.8% for boys and 5 and 7.6% for girls over this time period. Increases in dietary fat intake and lower levels of physical activity have been attributed to the increasing levels of obesity

— nutritional status of Kuwaiti elementary school children (6-10 years old) the level of obesity (defined as z-scores >2) was significantly higher for boys (15.7%) than girls (13.8%). Stunting was found to be higher in boys as well, 9.5% compared to 4.6% in girls. Obesity levels have increased significantly from 12.9% to 21.9% (above the 95 percentile weight-for-height) . In the US, 13% of similarly aged children (6 -11 years old) were above the 95 percentile These results indicate that Kuwaiti school children have a higher prevalence of obesity than US school children

— an urban low-income population in Brazil, although wasting (10.2%) was the most prevalent form of malnutrition, adolescent girls had stunting levels of 11%

and an obesity rate of 5.5%. Girls suffered more from stunting and overweight/obesity than boys did. These results suggest that improved living conditions in urban areas in populations 'adapted' to chronic food shortages may increase the susceptibility to obesity

— a representative study of 10 to 13 year old school children from both private and public schools in the urban area of San Jose, Costa Rica found that the prevalence of overweight was similar in both groups, with 31% overweight. These findings suggest that overweight is equally a problem among children from lower income families as among children from families with higher incomes

— in a cross sectional study of school children 9 to 16 years old from a low to middle income town in the Mexico City area, found that 24% of the children were obese. Television viewing was associated with an increased risk for obesity, a 12% greater risk for each additional hour of daily TV viewing was estimated. Participating in physical activity, particularly vigorous physical activity was found to protect against obesity; and

— a longitudinal study of 2,252 primary and secondary school children in Hat Yai, a urban area in Thailand, found that overweight in males increased from 12.4% in 1992 to 21% in 1997, however, the percentage of overweight in females decreased from 15.2% to 12.6%. Over the 5-year period of the study, children who were overweight during childhood were 12 times more likely to be overweight during adolescence than their non-overweight classmates. A family history of obesity, a monthly income greater than 5,000 baht, a low exercise level and one or more parents with high a BMI level were associated with overweight tracking. This study supports the importance of early intervention to prevent the persistence of overweight into adolescence and adulthood.

Short Term Hunger and School Nutrition Programmes (SNP)

There is increasing evidence of the negative consequences for children suffering from short term hunger, particularly in children who are not fed before going to school. Children who are hungry are more likely to have difficulty concentrating and performing complex tasks, even if otherwise well nourished. In recent years there has been some doubt about the value of stand-alone school feeding programmes in terms of their impact on either nutrition of education. However, the value when implemented in the right context should not be underestimated.

In 2000, a School Feeding/Food for Education stakeholders meeting brought together top practitioners and experts from USAID, USDA, the World Bank, UNICEF and other organizations who either administer or implement SNPs, who reviewed the current situation. Recent studies show the impact of what alleviating short term hunger can have on children's education:

— a project in Indonesia that piloted the integration of deworming with a SNP found that combining these interventions has an even greater impact on growth than when food alone was provided. In India, school children participating in a SNP were also provided with treatment for geohelminths. This resulted in a reduction in helminth infection from 71% to 40% with minimal additional costs

— an evaluation of a SNP in Jamaica examined the effects of the school meal on achievement, attendance and growth over a period of two semesters. It was found that the provision of breakfast resulted in higher school attendance and greater achievement in arithmetic although no weight gain was found

— Jamaica examined the effects in the short term on the cognitive function of children of differing nutritional status. It was found that cognitive function improved in undernourished children when they received breakfast while no difference was observed in well-nourished children

– providing breakfast only benefited children's classroom behaviour if they attended well equipped and organized schools. The behaviour of children in poorly organized schools given breakfast deteriorated.

Table 1. Morbidity and mortality associated with various water and sanitation related diseases.

Disease type	*Morbidity (no. of cases each year*	*Mortality (deaths each year)*
Diarrhoea	>4,000m	2.5m
Amoebic dysentery	48,000	70,000
Cholera145,000	10,000	
Roundworm	250m	60,000
Hookworm	151m	65,000
Whipworm	43.5m	10,000
Guinea worm	70,000	none
Trachoma	600m	none
Schistosomiasis	200,000	20,000

— in Mexico, evaluated the impact of a School Breakfast Programme. It examined the effects of school breakfast on the attention, memory and motor skills of 300 students, aged 4-6 years from impoverished areas. Children who received breakfast showed significant improvements in response, speed and fine motor skills when compared to the control group. Performance in verbal behaviour and short-term memory were not improved. The difference in these results as compared to other studies may be explained by the younger ages of the students in the study; and

— the impact of a mid day meal (MDM) programme in 60 primary schools in India. It reported significantly higher enrollment, attendance, and retention rates with reduced drop-out rates among MDM programme children.

Health Problems

The poor, particularly children in low income countries, carry the greatest burden of morbidity and mortality. Much of this burden results from hazards within their homes or their immediate environment. High levels of malnutrition, and its known synergistic relationship exacerbate their vulnerability to disease particularly diarrhoeal disease, helminth infections, acute respiratory infections (ARIs) and malaria. For the urban poor in low income countries, there is a double jeopardy as they find themselves exposed to both "traditional" diseases of poor sanitation and overcrowding and the "modern" diseases of chronic heart and lung disease. School-age children living in poor urban areas are also at a high risk of injury from road traffic accidents.

For children in low income countries, many of the health problems of childhood are associated with lack of clean water and poor sanitation (Table 1).

Diarrhoeal diseases

Diarrhoea is the passage of loose or liquid stools, more frequently than is normal for the individual. It is primarily a symptom of intestinal infection, cased by a wide range of viral, bacterial and parasitic organisms. One of the most common means of infection is through water contaminated with human faeces. If severe or persistent, the fluid loss and dehydration associated with diarrhoea may be life threatening, especially in infants and young children, the malnourished, or people with impaired immunity.

The total global number of diarrhoeal episodes may be as high as 4000m. WHO estimates that 3.3m children die from intestinal infections such as cholera, typhoid or infectious hepatitis every year. The total number of diarrhoeal episodes may be as high as 4000m (Table 1) . Most of the diarrhoeal disease burden occurs in children in developing countries, with underfives at greatest risk. Approximately 90% of the diarrhoeal disease burden is related to environmental factors of poor sanitation and lack of access to clean water and safe food. A recent review of 144 different interventions demonstrated the impact on morbidity of general water, sanitation and hygiene interventions:

— 36% median reduction of diarrhoea from the safe disposal of faeces

— 35% median reduction of diarrhoea from handwashing with soap after contact with stools

— 20% median reduction in diarrhoea from protection of water from faecal contamination; and

— 26% median reduction in diarrhoea from the integration of hygiene education or promotion in water projects.

Diarrhoea Prevention

Since inadequate access to clean water, lack of adequate sanitation facilities and poor hygienic practices are high risk transmission factors for diarrhoeal diseases, there has been increased emphasis on hygiene promotion programmes as a means of changing behaviour and reducing the incidence of diarrhoeal diseases.

— hygiene related behaviour in families in rural Nicaragua found a consistent relationship between almost all hygiene practices (hand washing, food handling hygiene, disposal of faeces, etc.) and incidence of diarrhoea, with an association between number of years of schooling and better hygiene behaviour

— in Burkina Faso, a study looked at a three-year programme of hygiene promotion behaviour, targeted at mothers of young children. The study found that mothers who had been in contact with the programme showed a significant increase in behaviours such as hand washing with soap after cleaning a child's bottom or using the latrine. The authors concluded that hygiene promotion programmes can change behaviour, and are more likely to be effective if sustained over time, using locally appropriate channels of communication; and

— a further approach to diarrhoea prevention has been examined in Pakistan. Flies are known to be a potential source of spreading diarrhoeal diseases, through contact with faeces and food. Although fly control has previously been classified as an ineffective prevention measure by WHO, villages treated with insecticide during the 'fly season' had an incidence of diarrhoea that was 23% lower than untreated villages. Although long term routine spraying is inappropriate, as a short term measure, selective fly control during the 'fly season' might be useful in some circumstances.

School Sanitation and Hygiene

Hygiene promotion in schools is a primary intervention because of the potential high risk of disease transmission if facilities are either non-existent, in a poor state of repair or incorrectly used. In addition, studies show that school-age children can provide effective links with their peers (child to child) and the wider community in communicating important hygiene messages as well as promoting improved sanitation. Encouraging safer behaviour through participatory hygiene promotion has been shown to be more effective than traditional didactic measures, especially when linked with parallel efforts promoting hygienic behaviour, safe water and sanitation projects within in the community. In many schools, facilities are either poor or absent.

The aim of any school sanitation, hygiene and water programme is to combine hardware and 'software'. The former revolves around the construction of facilities and their subsequent maintenance and use, while the latter focuses on necessary and appropriate learning experiences to encourage safe practice at school, home and throughout later life. As well as assisting with the construction, maintenance and cleaning of facilities in the school environment, studies reveal that promoting latrine construction through school children can be a successful medium for promoting construction in the wider community.

Hygiene promotion is now seen as an intrinsic element of any water and sanitation initiative and, in the context of school health, is now a central focus for school sanitation and hygiene programme. This approach has the following key elements:

— the safe, efficient and hygienic disposal of faeces, particularly child faeces

— the safe, efficient and hygienic management of water, from extraction, through transport and storage to use (particularly for drinking and hand-washing); and

— the regular and effective use of water (with a scouring agent like soap or ash) for hand-washing after contact with stools.

These three are generally considered to be the most important behavioural domains because they carry the greatest potential risk both on a personal and a communal level. There is increasing recognition of the importance of promoting safe hygiene behaviour among school children not simply because of its importance in the immediate school environment but also because of the communication opportunities and potential influence on the family and future families.

In addition to the obvious health benefits and time savings (particularly affecting young school-age girls), such programmes can also have an influence on school enrollment and attendance. The lack of adequate, separate sanitary facilities in schools is one of the main factors preventing girls from attending school, particularly when menstruating.

— in Bangladesh, a school sanitation programme increased girls' enrollment by 11%, a level that is beyond the reach of conventional educational reform.

Helminth Infections

Parasitic helminth infections are a major public health problem throughout the world with over a quarter of the world's population infected with one or more of the most common of these parasites: roundworm (Ascaris lumbricoides), whipworm (Trichuris trichiura) and hookworm (Necator americanus and Ancylostoma duodenale); and the schistosomes: Schistosoma haematobium (urinary) and S. mansoni and S. japonicum (intestinal)

Infection with intestinal worms is by a simple faecal-oral route. Infection with schistosomes is through contact with contaminated water (e.g. wading, bathing or swimming in ponds, rivers or lakes) that also contains fresh water snails that act as intermediate hosts.

Prevalence of these infections rises to a maximum in childhood and settles to a stable asymptote in the adult population. However, for the age-intensity (or worm burden) profile, there is a marked convexity, such that it is the school-age child who has the most intense infections (the greatest worm burden). As morbidity is directly related to the intensity of infection, it follows that it is this age group who is particularly susceptible. A similar picture is seen for Schistosoma age-infection patterns.

Helminth Infections in the Schoolage Child

It is estimated that over 35% (320m) of school-age children are infected with roundworm; 25% (233m) with whipworm and 26% (239m) with hookworm. As the intensity of infection is the central determinant of the severity of morbidity, it is the school-age child who is most at risk; for girls and boys aged 5-14 years in low income countries, intestinal worms alone account for an estimated 12 and 11% respectively of the total disease burden of this age group, making this the single largest contributor to the disease burden of this group.

As numbers of worms build up over time, many of the health problems caused by these worms are chronic and can be long lasting. In addition polyparasitism is a common occurrence; children may be infected concurrently with several parasite species. Children with chronic worm infections and large numbers of worms may be stunted and underweight, which can lead to long term retardation of mental and physical development, even death in severe cases.

Worms can also contribute to malnutrition through inappetance and malabsorption and aneamia through loss of blood. The most significant infection causing blood loss is hookworm infection. This may be caused by blood lose at the site of feeding; exacerbation of bleeding by the secretion of an anticoagulant; interference of uptake of iron in the duodenum; impaired appetite (with moderate to heavy infections).

— data show a relationship between infection intensity and haemoglobin levels: as infection intensity increases (as indicated by an increase in egg output, i.e. eggs/gram of faeces), haemoglobin levels decrease

— school children in East Africa suggests that the degree of IDA caused by hookworm infection depends not only on the intensity and duration of infection and iron stores of those infected but also on the species of hookworm. Ancylostoma duodenale was found to be more important in the prevalence of IDA than Necator americanus.

The school-age child, but also pregnant women and preschool children, are most at risk from hookworm attributable anaemia. Attributable fraction analyzes indicate:

— for the preschool children: the anaemia of 14% of infected children and 28% of heavily infected children was attributable to hookworm infection

— among school-age children, the proportion of anaemia attributable to hookworm infection in all cases of iron deficiency anaemia in school-age children was 41% increasing to 57% for moderate to severe anaemia; and

— a study estimating the percent of cases attributable to hookworm infection in pregnant women estimated that

29% of all anaemia and 41% of moderate to severe anaemia was caused by hookworm infection. Whipworms can cause a degree of blood loss as a result of dysentery and mucosal damage, although it is likely that this is only of significance in severe infections. An association has been shown between anaemia and the roundworm, although how this is facilitated in unclear - possibly through malabsorption or inappetance.

Schistosoma infections can also lead to blood loss. S. haematobium eggs reach the external environment by being pushed from capillary vessels surrounding the bladder through into the bladder lumen, being subsequently released with host urine (S. mansoni eggs via the intestine). This activity leads to tissue damage and blood loss.

However, there has been uncertainty about the effect of S. haematobium on anaemia. Studies have shown that infection with S. haematobium can cause blood loss although it has not been clear whether, at a population level, this causes reduced haemoglobin concentrations.

Multiple infections (polyparasitism) in school-age children make the study of this relationship particularly difficult.

— in urban and rural areas of Tanzania compared the importance of S. haematobium and hookworm infections as a cause of anaemia in school-age children (7-12 years). The majority of children were infected with helminths, suffered from anaemia, were infected with malaria and were malnourished.

The study found that although infection with S. haematobium per se was not significantly associated with anaemia in children with heavy infections, approximately one third of anaemia could be attributed to the parasite. Many studies have focused on the comparison of the prevalence and intensity of schistosomiasis between enrolled and non-enrolled children.

— in Egypt found that the prevalence of infections with S. haematobium and S. mansoni were higher in non-enrolled school-age children.

— in Nigeria showed that although more out of- school children were infected than those in school, the difference was not statistically significant.

— in Zanzibar showed that non-enrolled children had a higher proportion of heavy intensity infections which were twice that of enrolled school-age children

— in Ghana, it was shown that adolescent nonenrolled boys were more heavily infected with S. haematobium than their school-going counterparts; and

— in Tanzania, however, did not find any difference in the prevalence of parasitic infections between enrolled and non-enrolled school children, but non-enrolled children were more stunted, wasted and anaemic.

The hypothesis that non-enrolled children may have worse health than children in school may be true for some indicators of health status, but that consistently finding worse health cannot be expected.

Impact of Helminth Infections on Education

Establishing the linkages between helminth infection and cognitive development in school-age children is complex. Several studies have shown that children with moderate to heavy parasitic helminth infections are associated with lower tests cores of cognitive function and of educational achievement. However, convincing evidence of a causal link between helminth infection and cognitive function is yet to emerge.

— in a recent cross-study of school children that controlled for biological, socioeconomic and educations factors, helminth infection was associated with cognitive impairment. Children with heavy S. haematobium infections had significantly lower scores than uninfected children on short term memory and reaction time tests

— the major studies into the effects of helminth infection on cognition concluded that although the majority of studies have demonstrated an association, many of these studies are notable to conclude whether cognitive impairment is actually caused by infection or simply co-occurs with it

— randomized treatment trials concluded that there was no evidence of improvement in cognitive function following deworming

— however, treatment does appear to improve cognitive development in children who suffer from the heaviest parasitic loads and who are undernourished; and

— a more recent helminth treatment study in Tanzania, implemented new cognitive measures of learning ability rather than measuring developed cognitive skills. The study showed that treatment did not result in immediate improvement. However when children were both treated and taught how to do the tests, their performance improved significantly more than children who were taught but not treated. These results suggest that removing the causes do not necessarily remove the symptoms; in addition to treatment, affected children may require remedial stimulation to catch up.

Control of Helminth Infections

Improved sanitation and hygiene provides the long term solution to controlling helminth infection. However, evidence showing the negative impact of helminth infections and the recent development of inexpensive drugs has led to an increase in mass control programmes. However, helminth infections are not necessarily evenly distributed, however. A recent analysis of prevalence surveys in Africa has found that the distribution of schisto some infection is largely independent of the distribution of geohelminths. This highlights the need for a cautious approach to combined control in areas where one infection is much lower in prevalence than another.

The expected benefical effects of de-worming include improved growth, appetitie, fitness, cognitive performance and iron stores. Recent information also suggests that deworming can contribute to the reduction of VAD. The precise mechanisms by which these improvements occur, however, are unclear.

Treating helminth infections may have become more critical with recent evidence suggesting that the chronic immune activation caused by helminth infections makes the host more susceptible to HIV infection and enable the virus to replicate more rapidly. Evidence also suggests that chronic helminth infections may account for the higher prevalence of tuberculosis in low income countries and may compromise the development of protective immunity upon vaccination. However, this is an area of controversy and is currently under debate. Deworming may also improve school attendance.

Treating helminth infection on school attendance, within six months there were significant improvements in attendance that continued for the study duration of 2 years. Due to the impact of mass treatment on the transmission of infection, untreated children (attending treatment schools) had improved attendance as well.

The effect of de-worming on growth have, as with previous studies, reported varied impact. Research suggests helminth infection suppress children's appetites and that treatment results in weight gains. However, improved height gains have not consistently occurred in treatment trials. The intensity of infection, the regularity and duration of treatment and nutritional status have all been identified as important factors that influence programme impact. Overall the growth and nutritional deficits caused by these infections have been shown to be reversible through appropriate treatment.

In Guatemala, school children who were given two treatments for very high levels of Ascaris infection (91%) were found to have modest increases in weight gain 6 months after the initial treatment a more recent evaluation study from East Africa into the effect of a school-based de-worming programme on growth after one year found that linear growth improved in children who received twice or thrice yearly treatment. Children who were less stunted and who were younger (less than ten years) benefited the most in Venezuela, a study of the effect of monthly anthelmintic treatment on school children resulted in a significant decrease in the proportion of children who were at or below the 10th percentile for height/age and an increase in the proportion above the 50th percentile after one year. At follow-up, eight months after the treatment, 55% were re-infected with Ascaris.

Those with the highest rate of re-infection were found to be stunted or underweight children in a randomised, double-blinded control trial in Brazil of 353 school children, those with mild to moderate S. mansoni infections were randomly allocated to treatment or placebo group. One year later, treated boys had significantly higher measurements of weight, triceps skin fold thickness, mid arm circumference, arm muscle area, and body mass index than untreated boys.

These results indicate that, at least in boys, chronic S.mansomi infection even at low intensity is detrimental to shortterm growth and development a study from Indonesia that looked at the effect of treating Ascaris in school children did not find any beneficial effecton growth five months after treatment in a study that examined the effect of treatment for helminth infections on growth, appetite and physical activity in 149 Indonesian schoolboys, the treatment group was given a single dose of albendazole, measurements were taken at baseline and six months after treatment.

Results indicate that treatment for helminth infection may increase growth, appetite and activity level six months after treatment in areas where malnutrition and helminth infections are endemic. De-worming treatment is recommended every four to six months in endemic areas, thus improved growth six months after treatment is an important indicator of impact a recent study comparing the impact of twice yearly and thrice-yearly de-worming with no deworming on the iron status of school-age children found that the incidence of moderate and severe anaemia was significantly reduced in the twice yearly group by 23% and in the thrice-yearly group by 55%.

The programme impact, conferred the greatest benefit to those at the greatest risk from severe IDA-A case control study of school-age children in Tanzania found that a combined single dose treatment for schistosomiasis and Ascaris resulted in asignificantly reduced intensity of infection in almost half the treatment group. The greatest impact of the combined treatment was on children who were anaemic and heavily infected with hookworm in Tanzania, cross sectional studies involving anaemia evaluation and parasitological examination were implemented before and at 10 and 15 months following deworming of school children. The baseline study reported a high level of anaemia, 54%; attributable fraction analysis suggested that hookworm and schistosomiasis were responsible for 6% and 15% of anaemia cases, respectively. Fifteen months after de-worming (with albendazole and praziquantel), the prevalence of anaemia was reduced by a quarter and moderate to severe anaemia was reduced by nearly a half.

Analyzes from this findings, suggest that school-based deworming programs can prevent anaemia at a cost per case prevented over 15 months of between US $68 a study of school children in China and the Philippines treated for geohelminths and schistosomias is found a significant increase in haemoglobin levels in those who received a single dose of praziquantel; and Beasley's study conducted in urban and rural areas Tanzania found that although infection with S.haematobium per se was not significantly associated with anaemia in children with heavy infections approximately one third of anaemia could be attributed to the parasite.

These results lend weight to the argument of integrating control activities for schistosomiasis and helminths. Recent research shows that school based deworming programmes can reach out to those not enrolled in school and be effective a study in Zanzibar showed that when a good communication network is established between teachers, parents, siblings and friends of schoolage children that all children (irrespective of enrollment status) can easily, successfully and inexpensively be included in school based deworming campaigns in countries where schistosomiasis is endemic, such as in Egypt, it has been shown that interventions in schools may not only improve the health of school attendees, but also can be an affordable way of extending services to out of school children; and further research tested an intervention to extend routinely applied school-based treatment to out of school children and showed that out of schoolchildren can be reached at a relatively low cost.

Malaria

Malaria is probably the world's most important parasitic infectious disease, occurring in tropical and subtropical countries. It is caused by four species of Plasmodium parasite; P. falciparum, P. vivax, P. ovale and P.malariae. Several species of Anopheles mosquito can act as the definitive host, and it is transmitted via the bite of infected female mosquitoes, which breed in fresh (or occasionally brackish) water. The symptoms of malaria include fever, chills, headache, nausea, muscle aches, tiredness, vomiting, diarrhoea, anaemia and jaundice. In severe cases, it can also cause convulsions, coma, severe anaemia and kidney failure. Globally the malaria situation is serious and worsening with mortality ranging between 1.5-2.7m and morbidity 300-500m annually. Although malaria affects 40% of the world's population, 90% of the burden is in Africa (south of the Sahara).

Malaria in School-age Children

Most studies to date have focused primarily upon pre-schoolchildren estimating that over 75% of all-age malaria mortality is experienced by this age group. In contrast there are few empirical studies on mortality in school-aged children. However, recent preliminary estimates suggest mortality among school-aged children is between 5-14% lower than among younger children. This implies that malaria may still account for 10-20% of all-cause deaths among school-age children. School children who have not acquired exposure driven immunity may be at particularly high risk of severe and fatal consequences when exposed to the disease in unstable transmission areas. However, these risks are balanced by the low, and often very seasonal, exposure to the parasite. Pregnant schoolgirls are also a particular high-risk group.

Malaria is also an important cause of morbidity, but again, data is lacking, although recent data suggests that the risk of morbidity declines rapidly with age. Children aged 5-9 years experience between 0.25-2.3 malaria attacks per annum and children aged 10-20 years experience between 0.1-1.3 attacks per annum. Malaria can cause iron deficiency and anaemia. However, the effect of malaria on iron metabolism and anaemia is not fully understood, particularly in endemic are as where large numbers of school-age children are affected but are asymptomatic in a recent cross sectional study from Nigeria, 228 school-age children were evaluated to determine the effect of low-level plasmodial infections on anaemia.

The prevalence of anaemia increased when higher numbers of Plasmodium species were detected; and the prevalence of anaemia increased with the complexity and extent of Plasmodium species. These results suggest that low-level plasmodial infections also contribute to anaemia.

Impact of Malaria on Children's Education

Malaria accounts for between less than 3% and 8% of all reasons of absenteeism (0.001-0.021 days p.a.) . However, of preventable medical causes of absenteeism malaria counts for a significant 10-20% of school days missed per annum. Under the assumption that each malaria attack contributes two to five days absence from school, it is estimated that malaria is responsible for 4-10m school days lost (1% of all days lost in Kenya per annum) .The evidence also suggests that brain insult, as a consequence of cerebral malaria, in early childhood may have an effect on a child's cognitive and learning ability; residual neurological sequelae of 1-5% of children infected early in life.

The priority age group for malaria control is younger than school-age children. However, WHO and the World Bank are working with the Roll Back Malaria Partnership to identify an effective, operational response to the issue of malaria control in school-age children. Some interventions may be inappropriate for the school child. Kenya where the provision through schools of chemoprophylaxis, mass drug administration, selective treatment of infections and fever management with diagnostics were considered unaffordable options. However, school-based malaria prevention programmes are a good example of how schools can make a contribution to community health. It is suggested that children can be important agents for change in malaria control programmes.

The promotion, by schools, of prompt and effective presumptive treatment provides an affordable control option. Skills based health education can give children the ability to recognize the signs and symptoms of malaria, to recognize the need to seek treatment, and to differentiate symptomatic from curative treatment. Skills based health education through schools can also help promote a community wide understanding of malaria with particular emphasis on the need for community based control measures such as the use of impregnatedbed nets. Schools can serve as a focus for synchronised impregnation of bed nets and distribution.

Human Immunodeficiency Virus (HIV) /Acquired Immune Deficiency Syndrome (AIDS) and School-Age Children Approximately 40m people throughout the world are now living with HIV/AIDS (with 70% of these people living in sub-Saharan Africa), including almost 3m children under the age of 15. The impact and repercussions of this global epidemic in every sphere of people's lives is now becoming apparent.

HIV is a retro virus that attacks and weakens the immune system. Although an infected person may look and feel well for many years, as their immune system weakens they become unable to fight infection and become more vulnerable to a range of serious diseases, such as tuberculosis, pneumonia and cancer, and to opportunistic infections (such as fungal infections) that would not normally affect people with healthy immune systems. AIDS is the term used for the group of health problems, such as weight loss, various infections, tumours and other health problems associated with HIV infection.

HIV is contracted and spread through sexual contact (unprotected vaginal or anal sex); direct inoculation of with infected blood (e.g. through contaminated needles) and from an HIV positive mother to her child (at birth or through infected breast milk).

Prevalence in School-age Children

Throughout the world, HIV infection prevalence is lowest in the 5 to 14 year old age group, and AIDS mortality does not have its primary effect on schoolage children. The majority of children dying of AIDS are young children who have contracted the disease from mother-child transmission. An estimated 3.8m children have been infected with HIV since the epidemic began, and more than two-thirds have died.

UNAIDS estimates that in 2001, 800,000 children under the age of 15 became newly infected with HIV, and that 580,000 children under the age of 15 died of AIDS, the vast majority of them in Sub-Saharan Africa. During this time, approximately 2.4m adults (aged 15 to 49) died of AIDS.

Girls and young women are highly vulnerable to contracting HIV/AIDS for social, cultural, economic, and even physiological reasons. Alack of education increases this vulnerability, due to inequalities in status, power, and access to resources. Many girls and young women find that they have little choice and control over decisions about sex, and maybe exposed to unprotected sex, often with older men. This may be in exchange for gifts, money or favours, or as a result of abuse, including by teachers.

Direct and Indirect Effects of HIV/AIDS

Orphans and other vulnerable children The relatively low prevalence of HIV/AIDS in school-age children means that the direct effects of AIDS related illness in this age group constitute a relatively small proportion of the total burden of disease. In contrast, the indirect effects are enormous. Children may suffer both physically, socially and psychologically through death or illness of members of their family - including parents. In countries with the highest prevalence of HIV/AIDS, the concentration of AIDS in the working age adult population means that there are fewer adults to care for the increasing population of orphans and vulnerable children. This situation includes countries such as Botswana - where one in three adults are infected, Zimbabwe - where it is one in four, and countries such as Zambia and South Africa - where 20% of adults are infected.

One of the greatest impacts of the AIDS epidemic is on the children orphaned by AIDS. Before AIDS, anestimated 2% of children in Africa were orphans. Today, the proportion has risen to almost 15% of children in some African countries. It is estimated that 50% of these children were orphaned by AIDS. Over 13m children under the age of 15 have lost their mother or both parents to AIDS, most of them in sub-Saharan Africa. In less than 10 years time, the figure is expected to reach more than 25m.

Orphans are amongst the most vulnerable people in society. They suffer the trauma of seeing one or both parents becoming ill and dying from AIDS. Many will have to change home several times as they move to live with other family members or relatives, who may themselves become ill and die. They also run a greater risk of becoming stunted and malnourished and may miss out on schooling, due to lack of funds.

HIV/AIDS does not affect only households with children orphaned by AIDS; it also affects the children living with HIV-positive parents or relatives. This group of children serves as an indicator for the future orphan burden. The exact number is unknown and most countries have no estimates. Like the children who have lost their mothers or both parents, this group of children may be discriminated against, may lack basic health care and education, may experience physical and psychosocial stress, and may have little or no social and economic support.

The children are frequently young: the mean age of orphaning is only 6.2 years. They are also often forced to take on responsibilities far beyond their years, not only caring for other siblings but also for their parents - the people who they look to for love and support. An adult who has AIDS requires increasing help with everyday activities (which is expected from the child), but also suffers from frequent opportunistic infections such as uncontrollable episodes of diarrhoea, in conjunction with the slow debilitating effects of the HIV itself. The responsibility for caring for them frequently falls entirely on their young children. The psychological demands and effects on the child must not be underestimated.

Strategies to Protect and Assist Children

Children on the Brink 2002, outlines five key strategies for supporting orphans and other children affected by HIV/AIDS:

1. strengthen and support the capacity of families to protect and care for their children
2. mobilize and strengthen community-based responses
3. strengthen the capacity of children and young people to meet their own needs
4. ensure that governments develop appropriate policies, including legal and programmatic frameworks, as well as essential services for most vulnerable children; and
5. raise awareness within societies to create an environment that enables support for children affected by HIV/AIDS.

For school-age children, especially vulnerable children, finding strategies to keep them in school, or to reach them in out of school situations, is one of the key lines in defence against HIV/AIDS, especially for girls. By remaining in education, girls may have the opportunity to reduce the social and economic vulnerability that exposes them to the higher risk of contracting HIV.

Helping Orphans and other Vulnerable Children to Stay in School

Initiatives to increase the capacity of communities to support orphans and other vulnerable children have been adopted in a number of countries. Governments and NGOs work with the local community in a number of ways to support orphans and other vulnerable children, such as: offering community-based child care, allowing children caring for other siblings to attend school; persuading schools to accept more orphans; persuading guardians to send children to school; assisting vulnerable household with tasks such as tending crops or collecting fire wood. In Zimbabwe the government supports a Community Based Orphan Care Project, that uses community volunteers organized by local village committees. The volunteers help ensure that orphans are well fed, housed and clothed, and if possible attend and remain in school. Other countries to adopt this approach include Zambia, Malawi, Uganda and Kenya.

The major obstacles currently limiting orphans and other vulnerable children's access to education are: lack of finances; increased family responsibilities; discrimination, stigma and trauma; scepticism about the value of primary education and poor educational quality. A number of initiatives and proposals have been explored in Africa to try to overcome these obstacles:

— subsidy of prohibitive school-related expenses for individual children: In many cases school-related expenses, including textbooks, uniforms and PTA fees are more prohibitive than actual primary school enrollment fees. In some countries programmes have been initiated by local and international NGOs to help subsidize individual children or groups of children, often by linking them with sponsors or a sponsorship organisations. Countries including Zambia, Zimbabwe, Malawi and South Africa currently have such schemes, helping to increase access to school for some of the most vulnerable children, who are currently excluded for financial reasons. Community support and involvement is critical for identifying the most vulnerable children and families in need of assistance

— community schools: Community schools are run by the local community or churches. They do not charge fees and children are not required to wear uniforms. Local teachers are used, often on a voluntary basis. Such schools provide a more flexible approach to education, as timetables, days and terms of activity can be adjusted to local needs. Such schools are becoming increasingly popular in areas affected by AIDS, and have been adopted in a number of countries including Zambia, Uganda, Malawi, Mali and others; and

— distance learning and interactive radio education: Distance learning using media such as radio, is an increasing option for attempting to reach out-of-schoolchildren and youth. In Zambia a pilot project is under way in several Districts, using a radio-based learning system to reach students who do not attend formal schools. The pilot programme provides lessons in mathematics and English language, with students meeting for a limited number of hours each day in community centres. Trained, literate community mentors are matched with students to provide instructional support. Initial evaluation of the pilot programme has found it to be effective and popular.

Any strategies to assist children in gaining access to education should not be directed only to children orphaned 'biologically' by AIDS. They should be directed to all vulnerable children, who include children infected and affected by HIV/AIDS, street children, children exposed to strenuous labour, children with disabilities, children engaged in trafficking, and children affected by armed conflict. These children are sometimes more vulnerable than the orphans.

Psychological and emotional distress Besides the problems of adequate food, health care and education, an area that is too frequently neglected is the emotional distress of children living with a parent who is terminally ill, or who have lost one or both parents.

— one group that has sought to address this issue is the National Community of Women Living with AIDS (NACWOLA), in Uganda. They have started the' Memory Project', which aims to help HIV positive mothers prepare their children for the time when they will no longer be there to give them parental love, guidance and support. Central to the project is the 'memory book', prepared jointly by the mother and child, containing mementos, written pieces and pictures of family members and family life, together with advice to the children on how to live and take care of each other.

School-Based Prevention Programmes

Schools are the main institutions able to reach a large number of children and young people, with the support and involvement of the local community. Schools have the opportunity to reach children before they become sexually active, and while they are open to adopting healthy ways of behaving and protecting themselves from infection. Schools can serve as the forum where adolescents can obtain accurate information on reproductive health and HIV/AIDS, together with the skills and support needed to help them protect themselves from infection.

However, at present there is still little hard evidence that school HIV/AIDS prevention programmes that fail to adopt the skills-based approach have a major impact on sexual behaviour.

— a recent survey carried out in Botswana, Uganda and Malawi found that although the students in the survey schools were generally well informed about the causes and consequences of HIV/AIDS, this did not translate into major changes in behaviour. The researchers concluded that the economic, social and cultural pressures that led to unsafe sex amongst adolescents adolescents remained as high as ever. They found that teachers often received little or no training in HIV/AIDS education and lacked the confidence, competence and commitment to teach these topics. In many countries, school-based reproductive health and HIV/AIDS education is often used as part of a wider strategy of community and national HIV/AIDS prevention programmes, and may be most effective in this context, especially when a skills-based approach is utilized.

Skills-based Health Education

Skills based health education, including HIV/AIDS prevention, aims to help children develop the knowledge, attitudes, values, and skills- including interpersonal skills, critical and creative thinking, decision-making, and self awareness -needed to make sound health-related and social decisions.

According to major reviews covering 23 studies in the United States; 53 studies in Europe, the United States, and elsewhere; and 37 studies in other countries, including in Asia and Latin America:

— school-based HIV/AIDS prevention adopting a life skills approach to health education is effective

— behaviour change is possible if programs focus on specific behavioural goals, provide sufficient training and support for teachers, and use an age-appropriate and gender-sensitive design; and

— programme impact occurs slowly and is significant, but not large. For example, AIDS prevention campaigns in Switzerland helped reduce the share of sexually active 17 year old boys from 65% in 1985 to 54% in 1997, while the share of sexually active 15 year old boys in the US fell from 33% in 1988 to 25% in 1995. Note, however, that for the worst affected countries and those with large populations, relatively small and slow changes in behaviour could save the lives of millions of children.

These studies are encouraging:

— a recent evaluation of an intensive, two-year, school-based health education programme in Uganda found that the share of students in their last year of primary school who reported being sexually active dropped from 42.9% in 1996 to 11.1% two years later. A control group exposed only to the national health education curriculum showed no significant decline during the same period; and

— effective life skills programs have also been shown to promote abstinence and help children and adolescents to delay first sex.

There is, however, still a lack of broad evidence on the success of the skills-based approach in Africa, and few cases of large scale implementation of programmes, underscoring the need for greater monitoring and evaluation of the impact of interventions in the continent most gravely affected by the epidemic. The UNAIDS Interagency Task Team (IATT) for HIV/AIDS is an initiative that seeks to share experiences among countries in sub-Saharan Africa with the intent to promote Education for All (EFA) and the Millennium Development Goals (MDG). In an attempt to document seeming good practice, the UNAIDS IATT have published a Source book of school based prevention programmes that summarizes 13 promising programmes from eight countries in sub-Saharan Africa. Programmes were evaluated (only in terms of content) against UNAIDS Content Evaluation Benchmarks.

This synthesis shows that a child's ability to attain heror his potential is directly related to the synergistic effect of good health, good nutrition and appropriate education. Improving the health and learning of school children through school-based nutrition and health programmes is not a new concept. However, many early programmes have been characterized as being heavily focused on disease prevention, being uncoordinated, lacking integration and poorly evaluated and disseminated. Most importantly, the traditional school nutrition and health programmes have been based in the better off schools and in urban centres. This situation appears to be rapidly improving as new policies and partnerships are being formulated which help ensure that programmes are socially progressive and specifically target the poor, girls and the most disadvantaged children.

This change in perspective is timely as countries and agencies seek to achieve Education for All (EFA) by 2015, and address the Millennium Development Goals (MDG) of Universal Basic Education and Gender Equality in Education Access. If every girl and boy is to be able to complete a basic education of good quality, then school nutrition and health programmes are essential to ensure that the poorest children, who suffer the most malnutrition and ill health, are also able to attend school.

In order to operationalize an effective response, education sectors need to develop an infrastructure and policy context for improving the nutrition and health of school children. A major step forward was taken when a framework to Focus Resources on Effective School Health (FRESH) was developed by UNESCO, WHO, UNICEF, Education International and the World Bank and launched at the World Education Forum in Dakar in April 2000. Partners also include WFP, The Partnership for Child Development, and Save the Children US.

The FRESH framework provides the context for effective implementation of access to health and nutrition services within school health programmes. School based health and nutrition services, such as food for education, micronutrient supplementation and deworming, are most effective when they are supported by other strategies. These strategies include policies to provide a non-discriminatory safe and secure environment, provision of safe water and sanitation, effective referral to external health service providers and links with the community. The FRESH framework provides this context by positioning access to health and nutrition services among four core components that should be made available together for all schools:

— health related school policies
— safe water and sanitation
— skills based health and nutrition education
— access to health and nutrition services

These core components of the FRESH framework require school-community partnerships as the supporting strategies for the success of school health and nutrition programmes. These include effective partnerships between the health and education sectors, teachers and health workers, schools and community groups and between the pupils and those responsible for implementing school health and nutrition programmes.

Focusing initially on these activities allows concerted action by the participating agencies, and will ensure consistent advice to country programmes and projects. Because of the focused and collaborative nature of this approach, FRESH has increased the number of countries able to implement school health components of child-friendly reforms, and helped ensure that these programmes go to scale. The focused actions are seen as a starting point to which other interventions may be added as appropriate.

The actions also contribute to existing agency initiatives. They are an essential component of the "health promoting schools" initiative of WHO and of the "child friendly" schools of UNICEF, as well as of many other global efforts to make schools effective, healthy, hygienic and safe. The FRESH framework specifically addresses the need for nutrition and health services in schools. School-based nutrition and health services are effective and cost-efficient provided that the services are simple, safe and familiar, and address problems that are prevalent and recognized as important within the community. For example, improving meal timing or providing snacks can address student hunger during school, which seriously constrains learning and contributes to poor school performance. Similarly, semi-annual or annual oral treatments can be an effective means of addressing micronutrient deficiencies and worm infections. With treatment of worms, micronutrient supplementation is a cost-effective and simple method of reducing certain vitamin deficiencies in school-age children. School officials delivering simple health services in schools can easily correct these basic, yet pervasive, health deficiencies.

Technical documents have been produced by the agency partners in support of the FRESH framework, including:

— rationales for the four core FRESH activities

— a School Health Tool kit for teachers and programme implementers; and

— Fresh and its role in the Achievement of Education for All.

These technical documents are based on the current experience of researchers, policy makers and school health programmers and represent the 'best practice' for school health and nutrition programming. As a result of concerted action by the participating agencies, national programmes using the Fresh framework have now been adopted by over 20 countries in sub-Saharan Africa, ultimately benefiting a target population of 45m school age children. These school nutrition and health programmes provide an infrastructure and a context for the education sector to deliver a wide range of specific interventions. Partnerships of agencies are currently working to support intervention in some key areas.

The 'Food for Education' initiative of WFP and partners is working globally to address some of the nutritional, health and educational problems of school-age children. The initiative aims to alleviate short term hunger, improve the quality of student's diets, deworm and motivate parents to enrol their children, especially girls, in school and encourage them to attend regularly. So far 80 managers from a total of 21 countries and 30 technical personnel have been trained and formed a Regional technical resource Team. Deworming activities within WFP supported school-feeding programmes have started in seven countries and reach 520,000 children. Activities in 14 other countries are being planned.

The 54 World Health Assembly's resolution set a global target of scaling up intervention to regularly treat 75% of school-age children (398m) at risk by 2010. To achieve this goal, WHO has taken the lead in developing a broad partnership that promotes the incorporation of deworming of school-age children into existing institutions and programmes, for both the education and health sectors.

The Partnership for Parasite Control (PPC) was launched in 2001, with the aim of mobilizing resources and promoting new synergy among public and private efforts for the control of soil-transmitted helminths and schistosomiasis at the global and national levels. Working with the World Food Programme (WFP), the Canadian International Development Agency and the World Bank, WHO in 2001 trained representatives of the ministries of health and education of 21 countries, and deworming programmes have already begun in 19 of the 41 endemic countries in Africa.

WHO and the World Bank are working with the Roll Back Malaria partnership to identify an effective operational response to the issue of malaria in school-age children. Positive experiences by governments and civil society (especially Save the Children, US, and AMREF) in Senegal, Mali and Kenya are contributing to the creation of a tool kit of promising practices for malaria in schools.

An initiative of the HIV/AIDS affected countries and the UNAIDS IATT for HIV/AIDS and Education calls for a multi-partner effort from countries, development partners, civil society and the private sector to promote high level understanding and leadership, and the development of effective national responses across the education sector. The initiative seeks to share experiences among countries in sub-Saharan Africa, and has two main objectives.

First, to promote EFA and the MDG, which will ensure that every girl and boy has access to quality education despite the impact of HIV/AIDS on the education system. Second, to strengthen the capacity of the education sector to respond with timely actions to prevent students and teachers from being infected with HIV. The initiative aims to support country actions throughout Africa, and was launched in Kenya in November 2002. As part of this activity, and as previously mentioned, a consortium of countries and agencies has summarized 13 promising programmes from eight countries in sub-Saharan Africa and published a "*Source book of School Based Prevention Programmes*". But countries and agencies are now working actively to ensure that poor nutrition and ill health no longer hold children back from what may be their only opportunity to receive an education.

Objective of the Nutrition Programme

The main objective of the nutrition programme is, to reduce mortality and morbidity and to improve functional efficiency and productivity of the weaker sections of the community and provide nutrition to children in the age group of 0 to 6 and to the pregnant and lactating mothers. School feeding programme, I.C.D.S. (Rural) and I.C.D.S. (Urban) these three schemes are being implemented to provide minimum nutritional requirements and allied facilities to the most vulnerable sections of the society i.e. children, pregnant women and nursing mothers.

The Nutrition Programme is implemented by the Women and Child Development Department through the Commissioner of I.C.D.S. and Director of Women and Child Welfare. The outlay for Ninth Five Year Plan 1997-2002, Actual

Expenditure for annual plan 1997-2001, outlay and anticipated expenditure for 2001-2002, outlay for Tenth Five Year Plan 2002-2007 and for Annual Plan 2002-2003 are see on next page.

School Feeding Programme

The main objective of the scheme is to improve nutritional and health status of school going children and to ensure better attendance in schools. The supplementary nutrition is provided to the children in the form of 'ready to eat' food packets called "Paushtik Ahar" which is prepared out of local materials like soya, flour, bengalgram, maize \ sugar\ vanaspati\ refined oil,etc. 150 ml. of whole milk (after boiling) is supplied as a substitute of "Paushtik Ahar" at places where primary dairy co-operative societies have agreed to supply milk regularly through out the year.

The scheme envisages provision of supplementary nutrition to primary school going children of standard I in multi-teacher schools and children of 1st to IVth Std. in single teacher schools in the age group 6-11 years in rural areas of the State. The programme has been extended to the children in 2nd to 4th Std. in multi-teacher schools in tribal area of the State. Each beneficiary school-going child is given 100 grams of "Paushtik Ahar"or 150 ml. of whole boiled milk or one boiled egg on all school days except Sundays, holidays and vacations i.e. on 20 days in a month or 200 days in a year.

Integrated Child Development Services Scheme Rural/ Urban Areas

Integrated Child Development Services Scheme sponsored by the Government of India provides a package of services to children below 6 years of age and to the pregnant women, nursing mothers and adult women group of 15-44. The components of the scheme are Supplementary Nutrition, Immunisation, Health Check-up, Referal Services, Nutrition and Health Education, Non-formal Education.

(Rs.in lakhs)

Sr. No.	Programme 1997-2002 Outlay	Ninth Five Year Plan 1997-2001 Actual Exp.	Annual Plan Outlay	Annual plan 2001-02 Anti. Exp.	Annual 2002-2003 Oulay	Tenth Five Plan 2002-2007 Outlay	Year Plan
1	2	3	4	5	6	7	8
Mahila & Balkalyan Dcpartment							
1.	School Feeding Programme	......	......	......	......	......	......
2.	Integrated Child Development						
	Services in Rural Areas, Dist	21000.00	17711.46	3551.01	3551.01	3990.92	5000.00
	State	......	803.02	2800.00	2800.00	1500.00	15000.00
3.	Integrated Child Development	1000.00	10.65	67.59	67.59	71.02	2000.00
	Services in Urban Slums, Dist						
	State	......	70.11	400.00	400.00	200.00	2976.00
	Total ...	22000.00	18595.24	6818.60	6818.60	5784.74	24976.00

There are 268 projects being implemented in the state out of the total of 320 talukas. Of these, 202 are rural 26 urban and 40 projects are in the tribal areas and 99 projects under World Bank assisted ICDS III programme.

An ICDS project comprises around 100 Anganwadis & Aanganwadi normally covers a population of 1000 in both rural and urban areas and 700 in tribal areas. Each anganwadi has one anganwadi worker and one helper. One anganwadi Superviser is appointed for every 17-20 anganwadis who generally supervises the working of the anganwadi.

Three types of feeding is provided in the ICDS Scheme.

(a) Wheat based supplementary food prepared from the wheat.

(b) Local feeding from cereals and pulses produced locally and

The foodgrains and other materials required for preparing supplementary nutritious food is supplied by Mahila Arthik Vikas Mahamandal to the anganwadis. The food value of 100 gms. of "nutritious food" is of about 10-12 gms. of protein with 350-400 calories. Each child beneficiary is given 100 gms. of "nutritious food" per day at the rate of Rs. 1.82 per benificiary. Pregnant and lactating mothers and severely malnourished children are, however, given larger supply of 200 gms. per day.

The Government of India has accepted the concept of Mini-Anganwadis suggested by Maharashtra. This is an attempt to reach the outlying padas in the ICDS blocks where the beneficiaries are at a distance from the ICDS block and are unable to come regularly to ICDS blocks for nutrition. Under the scheme, it is proposed that for clusters of 3-4 padas a local adolescent girl will be given the responsibility of supplying nutrition to beneficiaries. It is expected that the M.O. will visit these anganwadis at least once a month. The proposed outlay in the Tenth Five Year Plan is Rs.24976.00 lakh, out of which an outlay of Rs.5784.74 lakh is for Annual Plan 2002-2003.

Index